FAT NO MORE

FAT NO MORE

THE ANSWER FOR THE DANGEROUSLY
OVERWEIGHT

NORMAN B. ACKERMAN, M.D., Ph.D.

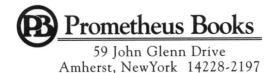

Prometheus Books
59 John Glenn Drive
Amherst, New York 14228-2197

Published 1999 by Prometheus Books

Inquiries should be addressed to
Prometheus Books, 59 John Glenn Drive, Amherst, New York 14228–2197.
VOICE: 716–691–0133, ext. 207. FAX: 716–564–2711.
WWW.PROMETHEUSBOOKS.COM

03 02 01 00 99   5 4 3 2 1

Library of Congress Cataloging-in-Publication Data

Ackerman, Norman B.
    Fat no more : the answer for the dangerously overweight / Norman B. Ackerman.
        p.   cm.
    Includes bibliographical references and index.
    ISBN 1–57392–692–2 (pbk. : alk. paper)
    1. Obesity—Surgery—Popular works. 2. Obesity—Treatment—Popular works. 3. Gastrointestinal system—Surgery—Popular works. 4. Jejunoileal bypass—Popular works. I. Title.
RD540.A25   1999
616.3'9806—dc21   99–17907
                                                                                    CIP

Printed in the United States of America on acid-free paper

This book is dedicated to the pioneers of surgery for obesity, especially Drs. Edward Mason, Howard Payne, Henry Buchwald, and others; to the many surgical residents who assisted me with the surgery and care of my patients; to the nurses and technicians in the operating room and patient floors; to the patients themselves, especially those who cooperated with me to try to achieve the most optimal result; and above all to my wife Anne who helped me at all phases in this work and in the preparation of this book.

All of the stories and anecdotes about my patients are true. I have refrained from using names or initials in order to avoid any embarrassment to the patients. But actually, there should be no embarrassment since I have tried to present these stories in a good light. These patients described are good people, but people with a serious problem. I hope I have helped them.

Contents

1

Beginnings

Eat not to dullness. Drink not to elevation.
—Benjamin Franklin

The year was 1971. I was director of the surgery department of a hospital in Kansas City, and I was on the phone with one of my surgery residents. He was saying, "Dr. Ackerman, there's a very fat man here in the surgery clinic. Why don't we do one of those operations that make the patients lose weight?" My reply, "No, I don't think so. I don't think there's any future in that kind of surgery." So much for being able to see the future! Or at least my future.

But after giving it some thought, I decided to learn more about these operations, and after doing so, I scheduled the patient for an intestinal bypass. I had a nice talk with the patient, Roger,* a man in his thirties who weighed about 340 pounds. I had never dealt with "morbidly obese" people before, although I certainly had seen many very, very heavy patients during my years of medical school and surgical residency training.

I remember one patient, Rachel, for example, who had an acute attack of gallbladder disease. She weighed about 250 pounds and was very short. After the acute attack subsided, she was told that we could not operate on her because of the added risk of infection and cardiac failure due to excessive weight, and we sent her home on a weight-reduction diet.

---

*All the names listed throughout the book are fictitious.

She was supposed to return to the hospital when she lost about 50 pounds. We never saw her again.

So, when I talked to this 340-pound man who seemed very ordinary except for his extreme weight, I wondered how he had become so heavy. I asked him to write down exactly what he ate at his three daily meals, for a period of about one or two weeks. When I looked at his completed list I was amazed. He was eating exactly what I was eating! A modest breakfast, a sandwich and a soft drink for lunch, and some meat and vegetables for supper. I'm about 5 feet 6 inches, and weigh about 150 pounds. I couldn't understand it. But as you'll see, I was pretty naive. A few days after his operation, while he was still in the hospital, I received an urgent telephone call from him. "Dr. Ackerman, come see me right away! I think I'm gonna die!" I jumped up and ran out of the hospital committee meeting I was attending, and ran upstairs to his hospital room. Expecting him to be slumped over in a coma, I was surprised to see him fat and pink with a big smile on his face. "What's the matter?" I gasped. "Look," he said, "I weigh 340 pounds. They're giving me Jell-O to eat. If I don't get a steak in me soon I know I'm gonna die!" And he said the word Jell-O with a very sick-looking face.

Well, this taught me something about the accuracy of the response of many obese individuals to the question "How much do you eat?" Later in this patient's hospital stay he informed the nurses that he usually drank a gallon of milk *with* his breakfast. Whole milk, that is, not skim milk. From this disclosure I learned that many people who are very heavy patients will tell nurses, orderlies, medical students, residents, or almost anyone else things about themselves that they will withhold from surgeons like me. So I look upon nurses, orderlies, and other healthcare professionals as my allies in the fight against morbid obesity. (Morbid obesity is explained later in chapter 2.)

This first case stimulated my interest in the surgical treatment of morbid obesity, an interest that has lasted more than twenty years. I saw these patients as not only an interesting medical challenge but as specific individuals who desperately needed help. There was nothing funny about them, in spite of all of the fat jokes, and the image of the fat, jolly person, which is for the most part an inaccurate myth.

Many of the hundreds of patients I've treated have asked me how I got into this field of surgery, expecting to hear some deeply moving story about someone close to me who had a similar problem. What I have just described is the real answer. There is nothing special in my background that made it inevitable that I would become interested in obesity and its treatment. I had a good education: undergraduate training at Harvard University, and medical school at the University of Pennsylvania. While in medical school I became interested in research, studying the workings of the thyroid gland. This could have led to a study of thyroid underactivity and obesity, but it didn't in my case. I continued to study thyroid function while I was an intern for one year at the Henry Ford Hospital in Detroit.

The following year I moved to Minneapolis and started my surgery training as a resident at the University of Minnesota. My research interest shifted from thyroid function to thyroid cancer, and then cancer in general. I studied the accumulation of radioactive phosphorus by various cancers, and developed potential diagnostic tests for several types of cancer, particularly stomach cancer. I wrote a thesis on my work, and was awarded a Ph.D. in surgery for my efforts.* As my cancer research evolved, I began to study the blood supply to various cancers, particularly the development and control of this circulation. I continued this line of research for many years, and I would like to think I have made some contributions to the understanding of cancer development and growth.

After I completed my residency training, I entered the army. I had been granted a deferment under a regulation called the Berry Plan, which allowed young doctors to finish their residency training before entering the military. I entered the army as a surgeon and spent almost two years doing surgical research on shock and blood circulation. After discharge, I began my career as an academic surgeon: I worked at Boston University Medical School teaching medical students and residents, operating on patients, and doing research and some administrative work.

During these early years after my residency training in the 1960s, various surgeons around the country were developing surgical techniques for the treatment of excessive obesity. I was unaware of some of this at first but I gradually heard more and more about it, though I never thought I would be involved with it. Interestingly enough, much of the most important work was done at the University of Minnesota after I left, or by surgeons previously trained there.

---

*This Ph.D. degree in surgery is not as rare as it sounds. Our surgery residency program in Minnesota encouraged us to spend some time doing research and most of us in the program wrote a thesis, took formal courses in pathology or physiology, passed two language exams, and defended our thesis at an oral exam, with the Ph.D. degree as a reward. The program was under the guidance of the world-famous surgeon Dr. Owen Wangensteen, and many major advances in surgery resulted from some of the research, including the beginnings of open-heart surgery and organ transplantation.

2

Morbid Obesity: A Definition

We must eat to live and live to eat.
—Henry Fielding, *The Miser*

The *morbidly obese* are those individuals who are at least 100 pounds over their ideal weight, and who already have, or who are likely to develop major medical or physical problems relating to their obesity.

This definition raises a number of questions. Why 100 pounds over ideal weight? What is ideal weight? What are the medical or physical problems? Why is it even necessary to have a special category such as morbid obesity, especially when "everyone" knows that being overweight is unhealthy?

First of all, there is nothing magical about starting morbid obesity at 100 pounds above ideal weight. I've been told that in some countries the definition of the term is at least 80 pounds over ideal weight. The point is that the patients who fall into this category are very excessively overweight, not just slightly chubby. I know of a surgeon who was sued by a patient who claimed that she was only 96 pounds overweight and was therefore not morbidly obese and should not have had an operation. This is nonsense! Even when one's weight is "stable" there are daily fluctuations of a few pounds, and on particular days this woman's weight could have ranged from 92 to 102 pounds over ideal weight. More important, even at 96 pounds beyond her ideal weight she is very massively obese and has all the potential risks to her health that someone 4 pounds heavier would also have. It's the spirit of the definition that is important, not being exactly 100 pounds overweight. Finally, as you will see, "ideal weight" is a somewhat complicated concept, and at best implies a weight range for someone at a particular height.

IDEAL WEIGHT

What, then, is *ideal weight*? To some extent it depends on where you are, and at what point in time, especially if we interpret the term to mean what we would ideally like to weigh and how we would like to look. In other words, it might depend on the ideal physical appearance currently in vogue. This has varied, to some extent, in the Western world throughout history. Obviously the beautiful women painted by Rubens and others of his period (sixteenth and seventeenth century) are much heavier than our present-day concepts of a beautiful, ideal appearance. Many other examples could be cited, and what we would now call somewhat overweight seemed to be a more desirable appearance in the past. This is also true in other non-Western parts of the world. Now, in the twentieth century, we have favored a slim, lean, thin, svelte, well-proportioned appearance in our men and women, and this has influenced our views of "ideal" weight.

At the present time, we often refer to the tables compiled by life insurance companies. These tables are based on their mortality data and represent ideal weights as those at which people live the longest. Such tables published in 1959 were used for many years, but a new set of tables was published by Metropolitan Life in 1983 (Fig. 1). In the newer tables the weights considered ideal are somewhat higher, particularly for the shortest men and women. There has been some criticism of these new figures and some physicians and others have still preferred to use the older tables. When you examine these tables you are struck by the realization that for any listed height there is a wide range of weights that may constitute "ideal" weight. A major consideration is the body frame or bone structure, listed as small, medium, or large. But even within the listing for each body frame there is a range of weights that is basically considered acceptable. As a result, according to these new tables a 5 foot 10 inch man could weigh anywhere between 144 and 180 pounds.

1983 Metropolitan Height & Weight Tables	1983 METROPOLITAN HEIGHT AND WEIGHT TABLES							
	MEN				**WOMEN**			
	Height Feet Inches	Small Frame	Medium Frame	Large Frame	Height Feet Inches	Small Frame	Medium Frame	Large Frame
Weights at ages 25-59 based on lowest mortality. Weight in pounds according to frame (in indoor clothing weighing 5 lbs. for men and 3 lbs. for women; shoes with 1" heels).	5 2	128-134	131-141	138-150	4 10	102-111	109-121	118-131
	5 3	130-136	133-143	140-153	4 11	103-113	111-123	120-134
	5 4	132-138	135-145	142-156	5 0	104-115	113-126	122-137
	5 5	134-140	137-148	144-160	5 1	106-118	115-129	125-140
	5 6	136-142	139-151	146-164	5 2	108-121	118-132	128-143
	5 7	138-145	142-154	149-168	5 3	111-124	121-135	131-147
	5 8	140-148	145-157	152-172	5 4	114-127	124-138	134-151
	5 9	142-151	148-160	155-176	5 5	117-130	127-141	137-155
	5 10	144-154	151-163	158-180	5 6	120-133	130-144	140-159
	5 11	146-157	154-166	161-184	5 7	123-136	133-147	143-163
Metropolitan Insurance Companies	6 0	149-160	157-170	164-188	5 8	126-139	136-150	146-167
	6 1	152-164	160-174	168-192	5 9	129-142	139-153	149-170
	6 2	155-168	164-178	172-197	5 10	132-145	142-156	152-173
Metropolitan Life Insurance Company Health and Safety Education Division	6 3	158-172	167-182	176-202	5 11	135-148	145-159	155-176
	6 4	162-176	171-187	181-207	6 0	138-151	148-162	158-179

Copyright 1983 Metropolitan Life Insurance Company   Source of basic data: 1979 Build Study, Society of Actuaries and Association of Life Insurance Medical Directors of America, 1980

Distributed as a public service by Lenox Hill Hospital

Fig. 1. 1983 Metropolitan height and weight tables. (Courtesy Metropolitan Life Insurance Company)

TECHNIQUES FOR MEASURING WEIGHT

There have been several other ways proposed for determining ideal weight that were to be used by all doctors. One of these is the *Body Mass Index* (BMI) in which weight (in kilograms) is divided by the height (in meters) squared. A 154-pound (70 kg) man who is 5 feet 10 inches (175 cm) tall would have a BMI of about 23. A BMI of 47 or higher is considered morbidly obese. A BMI of 25 or more indicates some degree of overweight. Incidentally, the BMI is also known as the Obesity Index or the Quetelet Index. Another way of measuring the BMI is to multiply your weight in pounds by 703, divide your height in inches, and then divide your height in inches again.

Other formulas that have been proposed include the Ponderal Index (height in centimeters divided by the cube root of the weight in kilograms) and the Broca Index (weight in kilograms minus height in centimeters minus 100). Other clinicians have used waist measurements, and waist-to-hip ratios as means of determining obesity. As you see, it can get complicated. Another problem is that some investigators feel that only considering height and weight does not necessarily indicate "fatness."

In order to try to measure fatness more directly, there are a number of techniques that measure the thickness of skin folds at the arms and other parts of the body using special calipers, a special measuring instrument. These techniques, which are called *anthropometry*, assume that the thickness in these areas of the body are representative of the fatness of the whole body.

To make matters even more complicated, there are other ways of measuring obesity that involve fairly sophisticated equipment and facilities that are not available to the average physician. Although interesting, these are mostly experimental, and include such things as underwater weighing, CAT scanning, confinement chamber methods, infrared spectroscopy, radioisotope measurements, neutron activation analysis, measurement of electrical activity, etc. As you can imagine, there is a fair amount of research activity on this subject.

Given all these attempts to understand and measure weight, how does one determine the appropriate weight for a patient and whether the patient is morbidly obese?

I still use a rather old set of formulas, but I find them the easiest to calculate and work with. I realize that my approach is not perfect, but after all, morbid obesity implies that the patient is *very* overweight, and accuracy to the exact pound is not necessary. In other words, if a person is approximately 100 pounds beyond what his or her weight should be, that's accurate enough.

The formula for ideal weight is:

Women: 100 pounds for a height of 5 feet, with an additional 5 pounds for each additional inch of height.

Men: 105 pounds for a height of 5 feet, with an additional 6 pounds for each additional inch of height.

Before you despair, a 10 percent range above or below your calculation should still be considered within the bounds of ideal weight. According to this calculation, I should weigh 141 pounds, but adding on the 10 percent (14 pounds), I'm fine at 150 pounds.

I realize that some people do have small body frames while others have large ones, therefore I refer to the Metropolitan Life tables if I have some doubts. But with the vast majority of my patients there is little doubt that they are morbidly obese.

OBESITY IN AMERICA

In the United States and much of the Western world, obesity is an extremely common problem. In fact, it is the most common nutritional problem we have. This is obviously not true in some parts of the world where famine, starvation, and protein deficiency are much more serious problems. But in the West, where food has become more plentiful, the incidence of obesity has soared.

There have been a number of surveys carried out in the United States during the last few decades that have attempted to document the actual prevalence of obesity. In a recent study by Kuczmarski and associates[1] covering the period from 1988 to 1991, 33.4 percent of American adults twenty years of age or older were estimated to be more than 20 percent overweight. This represented an increase of 8 percent compared with the survey done from the years 1976 to 1980. These increases occurred throughout the American population, although there was some variability depending on race, sex, and age. Another survey by the Harris Poll[2] indicated that 74 percent of Americans twenty-five years or older were overweight. Probably more than half of adult Americans are at least moderately overweight. Factors relating to weight gain may include inadequate levels of physical activity, decreased smoking, lack of awareness of actual food intake, and an increased consumption of food away from home.

There has been considerable interest in obesity in children. Factors in addition to those listed above would include physical inactivity (numbers of hours spent in front of a television set) and obesity in one or both parents.

Morbid obesity is much less common than being slightly overweight, but we are still talking about possibly between 4 and 10 million Americans.

The problem is greater in women, who experience obesity four times more often than men. There was one study by Lew and Garfinkel[3] that analyzed the weights of 750,000 men and women in the United States, and in the most obese category, women outnumbered men three or four to one. There is also a tendency to gain weight as we grow older, and this also appears to be more exaggerated in women than men. However, although obesity is more common in women than men, women may have a lower risk of developing medical problems and of dying as a result of their obesity. If true, this may be related to the general tendency in women of depositing their fat in the thighs and hips, rather than in the abdominal wall, which is the pattern supposedly more often seen in men. The theory is that abdominal wall fat is more "biologically active," having more receptors for hormones that break down and release fat into the bloodstream. While this may be true, morbid obesity is a serious threat to the health and well-being of all patients.

There also appears to be some relationship of obesity to social class, education, and race. One study in New York by Moore, Stunkard, and

Srole[4] noted that obesity was seven times more common in the lowest socioeconomic group than in the highest. Less-educated women tend to weigh more than better-educated women. Another study noted that black women in general are heavier than white women, but black men are thinner than white men. The study added that as they moved up the socioeconomic ladder, black men got heavier and black women became thinner. All of this may be due to dietary patterns in the various groups. There also may be some relationship to ethnic background. Americans of English, Scottish, and Irish descent are often thin. The tendency toward obesity is increased in those whose forebears came from eastern and southern Europe. While all the above is probably true, I should add that I have seen morbidly obese patients who are extremely well educated and wealthy; those in lower socioeconomic classes; males and females; and blacks, whites, and Hispanics. In other words, anyone can be morbidly obese.

There are other countries in the world in addition to the United States where morbid obesity is also a major problem. I am not aware of many studies from other countries that document the incidence of this problem, but there are surgeons in many of these countries who have had considerable experience in operating on morbidly obese patients. An incomplete list would include surgeons from the Scandinavian countries, Germany, France, Italy, Spain, eastern Europe, and Israel.

NOTES

1. R. J. Kuczmarski, K. M. Flegal, S. M. Campbell, and C. L. Johnson, "Prevalence of Overweight Among U.S. Adults," *JAMA* 272 (1994): 205–11.

2. "Three in Four Americans Overweight—Poll," Harris Poll survey mentioned in *New York Times*, 1993.

3. E. A. Lew and L. Garfinkel, "Variations in Mortality by Weight Among 750,000 Men and Women," *Journal of Chronic Diseases* 32 (1979): 563–76.

4. M. E. Moore, A. Stunkard, and L. Srole, "Social Class and Mental Illness," *JAMA* 181 (1962): 962–66.

3

Morbid Obesity: Past and Present

Let me have men about me who are fat;
Sleek-headed men, and such as sleep o' nights.
Yond Cassius has a lean and hungry look;
He thinks too much: such men are dangerous.
                          —Shakespeare, *Julius Caesar*

I have often been told that obesity, and particularly morbid obesity, is a condition of the twentieth century, or at the earliest the late nineteenth century. The implication is that only during the last one hundred years or so has food been plentiful and cheap enough for excessive overeating to occur. I don't believe this is totally correct. It certainly seems true that there is more obesity and morbid obesity than ever before. But all through history we can find examples of morbidly obese characters.

PREHISTORY

How far back? In my opinion, morbid obesity may go back to the prehistoric ages, specifically the Paleolithic period or Old Stone Age. In 1908, a 4.5-inch limestone statue of a woman was found dating back to 22,000 B.C.E. This is, I believe, one of the earliest representations of the human figure that has been uncovered. What's particularly interesting about this figure is its shape. There is a very round obese abdomen, large pendulous breasts, and very heavy thighs. In other words, this has the appearance of

18

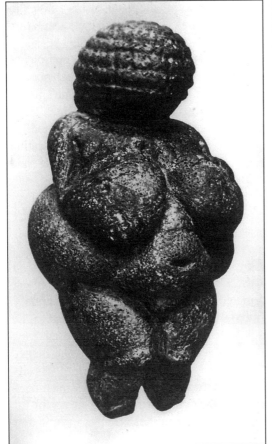

Fig. 2. Venus of Willendorf. (Art Resource, NY)

morbid obesity, and looks very much like our current patients. (That is, except for the lack of facial features and arms on the statue.) About a hundred other statues of this type have been found in prehistoric sites in central Europe, including Austria, Romania, Bulgaria, Yugoslavia, and the Ukraine. They have been called venuses, and the first one mentioned above is the Venus of Willendorf (Fig. 2).

Nobody really knows what they represent or why they are scattered around this geographic area. Among other things they have been called fertility symbols. However, the people living at the time when the venuses were carved were hunter-gatherers, not farmers, and fertility rites are usually associated with agricultural societies. There have been other interpretations. They may have been involved with the recognition of the importance of women's roles in the food-gathering process, most important in these ice age societies. Since many of the venuses have holes in them, they may have been worn as pendants. The definitive interpretation may never be known.

But, whatever their purpose, they are, in my view, representations of morbid obesity. I think they must have been modeled on real people. They're just too anatomically accurate to be the result of someone's imagination. They might possibly represent the chief's wife or daughter, since maybe they would be the only ones to have that much access to food.

Other obese female figures have been found. Caves in Malta dating from the Neolithic period, about 5,000 years ago, have these figures, and Egyptian and Assyro-Babylonian carved bas-reliefs are similar. The Maltese figures, made of clay or limestone, are in the Museum of Archeology in Valletta, Malta.

THE MIDDLE AGES

I don't recall seeing obesity depicted in ancient Greek or Roman statuary. But we are told that in the Middle Ages, Chisdal Abu-Yusuf was sent by Caliph Abd er-Rahman (911–961) to Navarre to cure its deposed King Leon of obesity. The treatment is not known but apparently he helped restore Leon to his throne of Navarre, according to E. N. Adler.[1] Obesity is rampant in the paintings of the Renaissance. Rubens, the Flemish master, painted many very obese, fleshy women, particularly heavy in the thighs and abdomen. There is a lush beauty in these figures even if they do not conform to our modern view of beauty.

There is other evidence of obesity in the Middle Ages. Suits of armor, for example. In various museums there are suits of armor belonging to knights or horsemen of extremely large proportions. I have seen armor of this dimension that belonged to King Henry VIII. Of course Henry VIII was known to be very heavy. His earliest suits of armor in 1515 showed him to be a slim young man. Those of 1520 and 1540 showed a progressive enlarging of his body. The armor of 1540 can only be described as huge. Supposedly, in one period of five years the waist measurement of his armor increased by 17 inches. At the end of his life he was unable to move about on his own because of his extreme weight, and a movable structure was built to allow him to get from room to room in his castle. He died at age fifty-five of the complications of extreme obesity, after having had several strokes.

FICTION

In the world's creative literature there are many examples of very obese characters. One of the most important characters from my point of view was the fat boy in Dickens's *Pickwick Papers*. His appearance and behavior were accurate descriptions of a fascinating syndrome that has been named the Pickwickian syndrome. Dickens was obviously a very careful observer of mankind. But more about that later in chapter 22.

Shakespeare was certainly a careful observer of the world around him. His character Sir John Falstaff was in every sense a classic example of morbid obesity. He was self-indulgent, lazy, and easily out of breath, but generally witty and good-humored. He was also a braggart, a liar, and a rogue. Prince Hal and others taunt him continuously about his weight. When we first meet him in *Henry IV*, Part 1, he asks Prince Hal what time of day it is. Hal replies, "Thou art so fat-witted, with drinking of old sack and unbuttoning thee after supper and sleeping upon benches after noon, that thou hast forgotten to demand that truly which thou wouldst truly know. Unless hours were cups of sack and minutes capons and clocks the tongues of bawds and dials the signs of leaping-houses and the blessed sun himself a fair hot wench in flame-coloured taffeta, I see no reason why thou shouldst be so superfluous to demand the time of day."

Falstaff is, at various times, called Sir Sack and Sugar, fat-kidneyed rascal, fat-guts, Sir John Paunch (he replies, "Indeed, I am not John of Gaunt."), round man, fat paunch, horseback-breaker, huge hill of flesh, a gross fat man, as fat as butter, and so on. Hal asks him how long it has been since he has been able to see his own knees. When sleeping, he is described "snorting like a horse," and Hal says "Hark, how hard he fetches breath." The Pickwickian syndrome several hundred years before Pickwick.

THE PAST FEW HUNDRED YEARS

There are occasional references to exceedingly obese real-life figures over the past few hundred years. A particularly delightful account is found in a small book entitled *The Life of Daniel Lambert—With an Account of Men Noted for Their Corpulence and Other Interesting Matter,* published in 1815. Daniel Lambert was born in Leister, England, in 1770. At age twenty-three, he weighed 448 pounds. He was very muscu-

Fig. 3. Daniel Lambert. (Reproduced by kind permission of the President and Council of the Royal College of Surgeons of England)

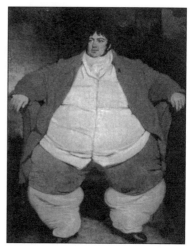

lar, could supposedly carry 500 pounds with ease, and was a good swimmer. He worked as keeper of the local prison. Naturally, Lambert attracted the curiosity of the local population. He decided to put himself on exhibition in London in 1806, and a special carriage had to be constructed for him for the trip to London. There, he was visited by "a great deal of the best company." There was no "indignity or insult from curiosity" but only "politeness and attention." There were many foreign visitors. Most memorable was a visit by a celebrated Polish dwarf, a meeting of the largest and the smallest.

Lambert returned to Leister after five months, and then traveled around England until June of 1809 when he suddenly died at age thirty-nine. His weight a few days before death was 739 pounds. He was 5 feet 11 inches tall and was measured at 3 yards 4 inches around his body and 1 yard 1 inch around his leg (Fig. 3). The coffin was 6 feet 4 inches long, 4 feet 4 inches wide, and 2 feet 4 inches deep. It took twenty men to lower the coffin into the earth.

According to this published account, he ate with moderation and his food differed in no respect from that of other men. The book concludes that "with respect to humanity, temperance, and liberality of sentiment, Lambert may be held up as a model worthy of general imitation."

In keeping with the title of the book, other very obese men were mentioned. John Lowe was originally thin, but gradually gained weight to 364 pounds. He "suffocated by fat," dying at age forty-one. A Mr. Palmer weighed 350 pounds, but appeared of "diminutive size" when he visited Daniel Lambert. Edward Bright weighed 144 pounds at age twelve and a half, 336 pounds at age twenty, 534 pounds a year before death, and an estimated 616 pounds at death. He was 5 feet 9 inches tall and 6 feet 11 inches around his abdomen. Bright was described as very strong, often riding horses, but of restricted activity because of shortness of breath at the end of his life. When he had an inflamed leg and fever, he was treated by bleeding, two pounds of blood at a time. He married at age twenty-two and had five children. His wife was pregnant with a sixth child at the time of Bright's death. Death occurred at age thirty of "miliary fever" (probably tuberculosis). It was said that seven men standing together could be buttoned in his coat.

THE NINETEENTH CENTURY

By the middle of the nineteenth century obesity and even morbid obesity were much more prevalent. It was felt that a stout, solid individual gave the impression of stability, security, and total reliability. Perhaps that is why so many of the leading politicians of the time were so heavy. U.S. presidents Zachary Taylor, Millard Fillmore, Ulysses S. Grant, and Chester A. Arthur were all described as "paunchy." Grover Cleveland weighed in at 250 pounds. A Pennsylvania political boss, Boies Penrose could not squeeze into a theater seat.

The largest of all was President William Howard Taft. Standing at 6 feet 2 inches, he weighed 275 pounds in 1900, 321 pounds in 1905, down to 250 pounds in 1906, and 355 pounds in 1909. He apparently became stuck in the White House bathtub on one memorable day. On a trip to Japan, the whole population of a village he visited turned out to help push him up a hill in his rickshaw. They had never seen anyone that heavy before. Times certainly have changed. Most American politicians try to maintain a slim, or at least nonobese, athletic-type appearance. But a few years ago the prime minister of New Zealand was heavy enough to require a gastric bypass for his morbid obesity.

When discussing turn-of-the-century overeating, the legendary Diamond Jim Brady must be mentioned. He supposedly weighed about 250 pounds. Considering how much he ate, he certainly deserves to be mentioned in this book. I will quote from James Trager's wonderful volume *The Food Book*:

> Brady's appetite and capacity defied belief. He was able to indulge that appetite by virtue of a lavish expense account.

For breakfast, Diamond Jim customarily had a gallon of orange juice (he had several beakers of it at every meal), hominy, eggs, corn bread, muffins, flapjacks, chops, fried potatoes and a beefsteak.

At eleven-thirty in the morning he had a snack: two to three dozen clams and oysters.

He lunched at twelve-thirty: more oysters and clams, two or three deviled crabs, a brace of broiled lobsters, a joint of beef, salad and several kinds of pie. And more orange juice.

An afternoon tea consisted of a platter heaped with seafood, washed down with a few bottles of lemon soda.

Charles Rector's was a favorite place for dinner (Rector said Brady was the best twenty-five customers he had). A typical dinner for Diamond Jim began with two or three dozen Lynnhaven oysters, each six inches from tip to tail.

Crabs followed, six of them, eaten claws and all. Then came soup, green turtle soup as a rule, at least two bowls. Diamond Jim was just getting warmed up.

He went on to eat six or seven lobsters, two whole canvasback ducks, two portions of terrapin, a sirloin steak, vegetables and dessert. And when Diamond Jim pointed to a platter of assorted dessert pastries, he did not mean any special one: he meant the whole platter. He followed this delicious repast with a two-pound box of candy.

After dinner, Jim might go to the theater. And after theater, how about a bird and a bottle? Only for Brady it had to be several birds (game birds, shorebirds or wild fowl) and several bottles—not of wine (Jim Brady was abstemious) but of lemon soda. And maybe a little more orange juice.[2]

Brady lived this way for years, but eventually died at age fifty-six, allegedly of stomach trouble. (A comic of the day suggested it was due to all that orange juice.) At his autopsy, his stomach was reported to be six times as large as a normal stomach.

There are other interesting anecdotes. Barnum's Mammoth Lady in 1849 weighed 576 pounds. Another one, Rosina Delight Richardson in 1852 weighed 475 pounds. In 1865, a fire swept Barnum's Museum in New York. A tiger leapt from the second floor onto the city streets, escaped the policemen's bullets, but was killed by a fireman's axe. This fireman was so excited by these events that he ran headlong into the burning building and carried out to safety the fat lady who weighed more than 400 pounds.

THE TWENTIETH CENTURY

The early years of the movies had their share of obese actors and actresses. Most notable were Ed Dunkhorst, "The Human Freight Car," who played in a 1908 film called *The Fat Baby,* and Fatty Arbuckle (who I think said "Nobody loves a fat man"). In more recent years, we have seen plenty of excessive obesity in the movies (*What's Eating Gilbert Grape* and the wonderful German actress Marianne Sagebrecht), theater, opera, football fields, wrestling rings, weight-lifting competitions, track-and-field competitions, and so on. It's hard to get exact weights of most of these people, but morbid obesity is there. Opera singers have frequently been ridiculed because of their often imposing stature.

My favorite story concerns the beloved contralto Ernestine Schumann-Heink. I don't know how much she weighed at the time of this story, but she was quite heavy. As she walked from the back of the orchestra to the soloist's place near the conductor's podium during a rehearsal of the Detroit Symphony, she kept knocking over music stands and musicians. In desperation the conductor cried out, "Madame Schumann-Heink, why don't you walk sideways?" As she continued creating havoc she replied, "Maestro, can't you see I have no sideways?"

Writers continue to use interesting characters who are excessively obese. Think of the brilliant detective Nero Wolfe, who apparently weighed one-seventh of a ton. He stayed mostly in his brownstone house in New York City, growing orchids, eating and drinking, and solving mysteries. Dr. Gideon Fell, another homebound solver of mysteries, weighed 250 pounds.

This more or less brings us up to the present. Maybe the final words on this belong to the *Guinness Book of Records.* It lists thirteen men who weighed more than 900 pounds. Supposedly the heaviest man of all time was John Brower Minnoch, born in 1941. His story is interesting. He weighed 392 pounds in 1963, and was up to 975 pounds by 1976. In 1978 he suffered from heart and respiratory failure and was rushed to University Hospital in Seattle. It took thirteen people to move him. His weight was calculated at about 1,400 pounds. He improved, and on a 1,200-calorie diet for two years he was discharged from the hospital weighing only 476 pounds. A record-setting weight loss of about 924 pounds. But by October 1981 he had gained back 197 pounds. He died in September 1983 weighing more than 798 pounds. Incidentally, his wife weighed 110 pounds.

Walter Hudson was a familiar name in the New York City area. He weighed about 1,190 pounds at his peak. Hudson made the headlines in September 1987 when he became wedged in his bedroom doorway trying to get out. He was finally rescued by nine firemen. Weight loss by dieting followed, but he then died, still very obese.

Possibly the heaviest man alive is T. J. Albert Jackson who weighs 891 pounds. His measurements include a 120-inch chest, 116-inch waist, 70-inch thighs, and a 29.5-inch neck.

Possibly the heaviest woman alive, according to the 1995 *Guinness Book of Records*, is Rosalie Bradford. Her weight was estimated at 1,200 pounds in January 1987. She was hospitalized, and on a carefully controlled low-calorie diet her weight in February 1994 had decreased to 283 pounds.

Other impressive heavyweight dieters included Michael Hebranko whose weight dropped from 905 to 217 pounds in less than twenty-four months of dieting; Paul Kimelan who went from 487 to 130 pounds in 215 days; and Richard Stephens who in 157 days went from 467 to 305 pounds. An impressive female dieter was the circus fat lady Celesta Geyer, also known as Dolly Dimples. Her weight of 546 pounds dropped to 141 pounds. Also impressive were the McCrary twins who weighed 743 and 723 pounds.

As you can see, morbid obesity has its own history, including some figures familiar to us as Henry VIII, Falstaff, and Diamond Jim Brady. An effective therapy might have robbed us of these colorful characters. Therapy, described in chapter 7, would have had a major effect on these characters. The therapy certainly had a major effect on the patients that underwent the surgery.

NOTES

1. E. N. Adler, ed., *Jewish Travelers in the Middle Ages* (New York: Dover Publications, 1987), p. 22.

2. J. Trager, *The Food Book* (New York: Avon Books, 1970).

4

A Cross-Cultural View of Morbid Obesity

Mortality, behold and fear!
What a change of flesh is here!
—Francis Beaumont (on the tombs in Westminster Abbey)

It's been too convenient to consider obesity simply as a consequence of Western civilization. But obesity occurs in non-Western parts of the world—e.g., India, Africa, Asia—and the story is an interesting one.

Much of this is related to the availability of food and its distribution among populations. Food shortage has been part of the history of humankind from prehistoric times to the present. Virtually all societies have had periods of food shortage, and possibly half of all societies still have at least temporary shortages. Some of these problems are seasonal, while others are periodic, often depending on the adequacy of rainfall for crops. The Pima Indians of the southwestern United States had a long history of drought occurring at least every other year. Now that food is abundantly available to them, they suffer from widespread obesity and diabetes.

It has been suggested that in areas of the world where food shortages and famine are common, individuals with a genetic tendency toward obesity may have an advantage in terms of survival and reproduction. Those who are able to store energy in the form of fat during the good years may have enough reserve to survive the inevitable bad years. Others may succumb to starvation, malnutrition, and lack of resistance to infection, and their infant-mortality rates may be excessive. Successful completion of pregnancy and lactation may depend on the degree of the fat reserve in women in some parts of the world. So, fatness and fertility are considered highly desirable, and are found mainly in the upper socioeconomic classes in these societies.

Anthropologists Peter Brown and Melvin Konner from Emory University have written about the role of obesity in these societies.[1] For example, in Nigeria young Efik tribal girls were sent into seclusion for up to two years into fattening huts before their marriage. Those elites who could afford to use these facilities considered fatness as the major criterion of beauty. Fattening huts were also found in other parts of West Africa.

Brown and Konner wrote that there was a similar emphasis on fatness for girls at puberty among the Havasupai Indians in the American Southwest. If a girl was thin, a fat woman would place her foot on the girl's back to encourage fatness. Fat legs were considered an important element of beauty. This was also prevalent in the Tarahumara tribe of northern Mexico, and a good-looking woman was called a "beautiful thigh." Thin hips were "dog hips," an insult used by the Amhara people in Africa. A courting song of the Bemba tribe in South Africa has the following words: "Hello Mama, the beautiful one, let us go to town/You will be very fat, you girl, if you stay with me."

There is an interesting story related by Brown and Konner about health-education posters put up in a Zulu community near Durban, South Africa. This was part of an obesity-prevention campaign. One poster showed an obese woman and an overloaded truck with a flat tire. The caption read "Both carry too much weight." A second poster showed a thin woman sweeping up under a table near an obese woman who was using the table to support herself. This poster had the caption "Who do you prefer to look like?" The community unfortunately misinterpreted the messages. The obese woman in the first poster was seen as rich and happy since she was not only fat, but also had a truck overflowing with her belongings. The second poster was seen as showing a wealthy mistress supervising her underfed servant.

The above has emphasized the desirability in these societies of fatness and fertility in women. For men the situation is different. The physical attributes that appear to be most desired in men are a tall or moderately tall stature and a muscular physique. But there are some societies where large size and obesity are admired and are considered to symbolize economic success, political power, and social status. This is true among leaders in tribal New Guinea. Large body size may be related to the accessibility of food resources of these privileged leaders. In the

Bemba of South Africa obesity in men is not only indicative of economic success but is also felt to be a sign of the spiritual power to fend off sorcerer's attacks.

Even today in Tonga, a Polynesian island in the South Pacific, obesity in men remains a symbol of social status. Many are described as fat and jolly. The king of Tonga, the last absolute monarch in Polynesia, is an enormous man of 440 pounds, with a liking for French food. Apparently his size goes along with the power of his office.

The most spectacular occurrence of obesity, and often massive obesity in men, is in the Japanese sumo wrestlers. Several good books have been written on the subject, including those by Cuyler[2] and Long.[3] Sumo wrestling may have had its beginnings as early as in the Western Zhou dynasty in China (eleventh century B.C.E.). Wrestling in China and Japan in these early years was associated with religious ceremonial and courtly rites. Sumo wrestling, archery, and equestrian archery were the great ceremonial sports in annual tournaments at the courts.

But as Japan became involved in civil war between the great clans in the twelfth century, sumo became a military art. Victory in battle was sometimes determined by contests between individual samurai warriors, and skills in sumo wrestling, archery, and swordsmanship were used in declaring a winner. The importance of sumo wrestling as a martial art disappeared with the introduction of guns at the end of the sixteenth century.

As a result, "masterless samurai wrestlers" wandered through the Japanese countryside earning a living by competing in regional sumo wrestling contests. Because of the occasional associated violence, swordplay, and death, all types of sumo were banned for a short time in the mid-1600s. As a result, in 1684 strict rules and regulations were set up to eliminate the possibility of violence, and sumo wrestling again became acceptable. For the first time in its history, the holds and throws that could be used were specified, and regulations regarding the sumo ring were agreed upon. This began professional sumo wrestling as we know it today, with tournaments scheduled in Osaka, Kyoto, and Edo (Tokyo).

For most of its history, sumo wrestlers have been men. But in the middle of the eighteenth century in Edo, sumo wrestling bouts between women were part of the popular entertainment of the day. Many of the women were given suggestive names, such as Chichigahari (Big Tits), and sometimes the women were pitted against blind men, with much groping and grabbing. This was all stopped in 1873, and was outlawed in 1926. Sumo wrestling is the sport of large, often very obese men.

Where do these enormous men come from? Japan, as we have known it, has been a country of individuals short in stature, and slight in body build. Young potential sumo wrestlers must pass a physical examination before each tournament. For those under twenty-one years of age, the minimum height is 5 feet 6$\frac{1}{4}$ inches, and minimum weight is 154 pounds. For those over twenty-one years, minimum height is 5 feet 7$\frac{1}{2}$ inches, and minimum weight is 165 pounds. This isn't very big, but they grow and they grow. For a quick gain of weight for passing an exam, a young man may stuff himself with sweet potatoes and as much water as his stomach can hold. After the weighing in, regurgitation of this mass of food is common.

Groups of the wrestlers are banded together in one of the sumo "stables," and go through a vigorous training regime. The first and major meal of the day consists mainly of *chanko-nabe*. The wrestlers, having exercised for hours without eating, approach this meal with a voracious appetite. Chanko-nabe consists of meat or fish, malt, cabbage, spinach, onions, carrots, daikon radishes, shiitake mushrooms, tofu, soy sauce, rich stock, and a lot of sugar, cooked together in a great pot. Wrestlers may consume five or six bowlfuls of this high-caloric stew, with an equal amount of rice in addition. This is all washed down with massive quantities of beer and sake. The actual calorie count? Who knows, but obviously high. This is followed usually by a long afternoon nap. The inactivity after this large meal is felt to be an important factor in the shaping of the bulging sumo stomach.

We have all seen photographs of the enormous champion sumo wrestlers. But how large exactly are they? And are they morbidly obese? I have looked through the lists of *yokozuna* or grand-champion wrestlers, which is the highest rank in sumo wrestling. There were fifty-four names on this list which included height and peak weight of each wrestler plus dates of birth and death. The earliest name is from the late 1700s. Since there are only fifty-four wrestlers who had achieved this ranking since that time up to 1977 (the date of my list), this is obviously a very elite group.

The peak weights of these yokozuna wrestlers ranged from 231 to 372 pounds, with the average weight of 297 pounds. They were all very tall, for Japanese, ranging from 5 feet 6 inches to 6 feet 7 inches, with an average height of 6 feet 0 inches. Were they morbidly obese? By the criterion of at least 100 pounds over ideal weight, 45 of the 54 were clearly morbidly obese, and 9 were just slightly below. Don't get me wrong. All of the 9 were pretty heavy. The lightest wrestler was Wakanohana Kanji, 6 feet tall, who tipped the scales at only 231 pounds. In contrast, Azumafuji Kin'ichi, also 6 feet tall, weighed 372 pounds.

In 1989, there were three yokozuna wrestlers still active. The heaviest, Hokutoumi, is 6 feet 2 inches and weighed 448 pounds. The others were Onokuni, 5 feet 11 inches and 318 pounds, and Chiyonofuji, a mere 6 feet 0 inches and 270 pounds. Of the wrestlers that had not achieved the exalted status of yokozuna, some have been even heavier than those mentioned above.

Jesse Kuhaulua, known as Takamiyama in his sumo days, was Hawaiian. He wrestled mostly in the 1970s. He was 6 feet 3 inches tall and weighed nearly 400 pounds. The greatest excitement in recent years involved another Hawaiian, Salevaa Atisanoe, known as Konishiki. Konishiki is big. Or to be more accurate, he is the biggest! Possibly too big. When he won his first Emperor's Cup victory in November 1989, he weighed 490 pounds. He was as much as 576 pounds and certainly was, at least in terms of his weight, morbidly obese. But he is vigorous, lively, and active, defeating most of his competition. He married his Japanese sweetheart, a model weighing about a fifth of his weight, and whose waist is thinner than either of his legs.

A few years ago, Konishiki suffered several injuries that have hurt his career. A stool he was sitting on collapsed and he broke his tailbone. Later, he injured his leg. This also seemed to be related to his very excessive weight. In 1997, he announced his retirement. Although only thirty-three years old, he suffered from gout, stomach ulcers, and knee problems.

There is another American, known as Akebono, who is a current sumo champion. He is also very heavy.

Now since we have established that many of the sumo wrestlers are heavy enough to be considered morbidly obese, do they suffer from the same medical problems that plague the morbidly obese elsewhere in the world? This is not easy to answer. Many seem to retire from wrestling in their mid-thirties. Most of them try to decrease their weight after retirement. After all, the original gain of weight was due, artificially, to their conscious effort to increase their caloric intake. But there appears to be some tendency toward diabetes and heart disease, as well as problems in their lower joints, particularly the knees.

Do they have a shortened lifespan? The average yokozuna lived to the age of fifty-five years. Since this includes a time period of the late 1700s to the present, a fifty-five-year lifespan isn't bad. A study of wrestlers active in the 1920s showed an average lifespan of sixty-four years, which was longer than that of the male population at that time.

Are the sumo wrestlers different than other morbidly obese groups? Possibly yes. The factors may include their intense physical activity, their method of becoming obese including the specific diet, the absence of obviously inherited obesity, and their ratio of muscle mass to fatty tissue. Certainly they are one of the most interesting subsets of the morbid obesity world.

NOTES

1. P. J. Brown and M. Konner, "Anthropological Perspective on Obesity," in R. J. Wurtman and J. J. Wurtman, *Human Obesity* (New York: New York Academy of Sciences, 1987): 29–46.

2. P. L. Cuyler, *Sumo: From Rite to Sport* (New York: Weatherhill, 1979).

3. W. Long, *Sumo: A Pocket Guide* (Rutland, Vt.: Charles E. Tuttle, 1989).

5

How Do People Become Morbidly Obese?

He hath eaten me out of house and home.
—Shakespeare, *Henry IV,* Part 2

Many people I know, including doctors and nurses, ask me, "How can people get so incredibly fat?" The answer is not as straightforward as one might think. First of all, there has been a lot of talk for many years about obesity resulting from "glandular" problems. While there are some endocrine or glandular abnormalities that can cause obesity, the actual occurrence of morbid obesity as a result of these problems is very uncommon. For example, an underactive thyroid gland or an overactive adrenal gland may cause someone to be overweight, but usually not heavy enough to be considered morbidly obese. Through the years I have seen only three morbidly obese patients with thyroid abnormalities. Two had underactive glands and when they were treated with appropriate thyroid medication, they lost 15 pounds. But they were still more than 100 pounds overweight. I operated on both of them with good results. The third patient had an overactive thyroid, and when that was corrected she *gained* 15 pounds. She also underwent surgery at a later date.

I remember seeing a cartoon showing a doctor talking to a very heavy patient. "Yes, you can consider it a glandular problem," he was saying, "if you consider your mouth a gland."

There does seem to be some question in the minds of various medical authorities about the amount of calories consumed by morbidly obese patients. Some, including Wooley, Wooley, and Dyrenforth,[1] claim that the obese eat no more than thinner individuals but these unfortunate obese people have a small "regulatory error." In other words, for some reason they burn off fewer calories than thinner people. While this is an attractive theory, there doesn't seem to be any way to measure this regulatory factor, at least at the present time.

Other authorities, including Payne[2] and Drenick,[3] feel that the problem is more straightforward. Massive obesity, they say, is due to massive overeating. While assessing caloric intake of morbidly obese patients may often be difficult and inaccurate, I have seen various studies, including that of Drenick[4] and Bray and associates,[5] suggesting that the average daily calorie consumption of these patients is anywhere from 2,500 to 7,000 calories. One surgeon used to talk about one of his patients who supposedly ate 15,000 calories a day.

Studies performed on my patients by a very good research dietician appear to confirm the overeating theory. The average daily caloric intake was about 6,500 calories, with 700 grams of carbohydrates, 215 grams of protein, and about 300 grams of fat. This is all far higher than our basic daily caloric requirements, which, depending on age, sex, and physical activity level, may range from 1,500 to 3,500 calories per day. I'll refer to the figures in my study later to compare them with the changes in eating habits that occur after the various operations.

I think the results in these studies are quite realistic. There are some research studies, including those discussed by Drenick,[6] showing that people weighing 350 to 450 pounds must eat more than 6,000 calories per day just to stay at that weight level. Every surgeon I know who is interested in morbid obesity can tell stories about the tremendous appetites of his or her patients. For example, one of my patients used to be invited every year to a Salvation Army picnic in her town. Everyone else invited was told to come a half hour earlier so they could get a head start eating. My patient arrived a half hour later when the others had finished eating, and according to several witnesses, the person would "clean everything up." What they meant was that she would eat absolutely everything that was left, regardless of the amount. She weighed over 400 pounds.

Most Americans are unaware of exactly how many calories are in the foods they eat. A four-ounce muffin may have 430 calories; 4 large unbuttered, unsyruped pancakes may have 610 calories; and a large tuna salad sandwich may have over 700 calories. Then there's pizza, french fries, hamburgers, steak, and so on. The tendency to ingest more fat-free and sugar-free foods has not helped, since the calorie count for these foods is still often too high.

My feeling remains that morbid obesity is for the most part due to massive overeating. But I have had patients who claim that they really don't eat very much. While I am not sure I believe them, possibly some people have this "regulatory error" that causes obesity. Let's keep an open but skeptical mind. (The good news is that virtually all patients lose weight after the operations, regardless of the cause of their morbid obesity.)

If we are willing to accept that most morbidly obese patients are that way because of massive overeating, the next question is an obvious one: why do they eat so much? Is it hereditary, environmental, psychological, or something else entirely?

It can be very hard to separate these factors. Several years back, I operated on a mother and three daughters, all were morbidly obese. It would seem that this common problem was hereditary, right? But this very nice family was extremely food-oriented. Their friends told me that the moment people walk into their house they are besieged by food. "Have a piece of candy." "Have some fruit." "How about some potato chips?" Bowls of food were everywhere. So was it hereditary, environmental, psychological, or some other cause?

There have been a number of good statistical studies, including those by Stunkard, Foch, and Hrubec[7] and Scuro and Bosello,[8] that have attempted to determine the role of heredity in obesity. One classical method for this type of investigation involves the comparison of findings in identical and fraternal twins. What is looked for is a similarity in the weight levels, either thin or fat, in the twins, or a lack of similarity. This is called a "concordance rate." This similarity, or concordance, is measured in identical twins, since they are genetically the same, compared to fraternal twins, who are not.

While some of the studies are of questionable significance, some very convincing ones, including those by Stunkard and associates[9] and Scuro and Bosello,[10] strongly suggest the importance of genetic influences in human obesity. One such study, for example, involved the comparison of several thousand male twins, using height and weight measurements when they were inducted into the military, and then similar measurements obtained twenty-five years later. Concordance rates were much higher in the identical twins, at all degrees of obesity, than the rates in the fraternal twins.

There have been recent reports in the *New York Times* of the identification by Dr. Jeffrey Friedman in certain genetically obese mice of a defective gene that might be responsible for the obesity.[11] The researchers theorize that this gene, acting on fat cells, produces a substance called *leptin* which, when reaching the brain, controls appetite. If the gene is defective, the brain is fooled into thinking that there is not enough fat in the body, and the intake of more food is encouraged. Five mutant genes, according to the article in the *New York Times* by Wade, are now known to affect body weight in mice.[12] Much additional research is needed before definitive answers can be found. Of greater significance is the need to determine the importance of this genetic component in human obesity. This research is exciting and we look forward to further work in this area.

While my own clinical observations lack the scientific or statistical rigor of a sustained study, I certainly have seen a great number of patients with strong family histories of obesity. Sometimes the patient will say that all relatives on the mother's side of the family are very heavy, but all are thin on the father's side. Or vice versa. Of course the same question of heredity versus environment keeps popping up. While it has been pointed out that obese parents tend to have obese children, this trend toward obesity also holds true for adopted children. And also for their pets! No doubt both heredity and environment are important.

Occasionally I'll see a patient who states that everyone else in the family is thin. Why then is this patient morbidly obese? The answers are not simple. There may be individual factors in each patient's life that have influenced lifestyle and eating habits. Sometimes there has been major food deprivation in the patient's childhood, and food, now available, has become a dominant factor, a symbol of success and survival. Some older patients have talked about the Great Depression, and how their family suffered from severe food shortages. I have also had several patients who were Holocaust survivors for whom food is a symbol of life itself. But most Depression and Holocaust survivors are not morbidly obese. What is different about those that are morbidly obese?

There are many other questions that could be asked. Many patients have been obese all their lives, starting in early childhood. Others started to put on significant weight later on, at specific times in their life. Obesity starting during adolescence is common. Many women have noted that they were thin until pregnancy occurred, and that they were never able to lose the weight that was put on at that time. All of this suggests endocrine or glandular factors, but what specifically are they?

Another common pattern is the "vicious cycle pattern." The patients are fat and the world is rejecting them. Personal relationships, education, employment, and the like are all unsatisfactory because of the person's obesity, or at least that's the way they see it. Only eating makes them feel better, so they eat and eat and eat. They become more obese and more depressed, and the vicious cycle goes on. This brings up the emotional and psychological aspects of morbid obesity.

The commonly held belief by most doctors and lay people is that anyone who weighs 300 or 400 or 500 pounds must be emotionally or psychologically sick. "Otherwise how could they let themselves get to that state?" Amazingly enough, there is no real evidence to support this belief. As a group, there are no major psychological differences between obese and nonobese people, according to numerous studies on this subject. One such study, authored by Dr. Katherine Halmi,[13] a psychiatrist, concludes that there is no evidence of an increased prevalence of major psychiatric disorder in obese persons, when strictly defined diagnostic criteria are used. However, there is at least one study, such as that of Gentry, Halverson, and Heisler,[14] that reported that the incidence of emotional disturbance was somewhat higher in the obese group studied than in people of normal weight. And, surprisingly, another study by Crisp and McGuiness[15] reported that the incidence of anxiety and depression were actually lower in their overweight group.

Such factors as eating under stress, being stimulated to eat by the sight or smell of food, and eating especially fast or slow do not appear to be more common in obese people as compared to the nonobese. Internal cues to hunger did not differ in obese persons from others in the studies of Parham, Keng, and Mohiuddin.[16] Other studies such as that by Lanzisera and colleagues[17] have concluded that the morbidly obese are a psychologically heterogenous or mixed group without any specific emotional factors responsible for the development of their obesity. At most, there may be some tendency toward being passively dependent, and according to the study from Washington University of St. Louis by Gentry, Halverson, and Heisler,[18] with more depressive traits and less self-esteem. These are hardly major factors. Now having said all of this, one must admit that some obese patients individually do seem to suffer from major psychological problems that relate to their weight problem. However, there does not appear to be an "obesity psychological trait" responsible for the development of morbid obesity.

Finally, there are probably important social and perhaps ethnic factors involved. Food and eating are sometimes overemphasized in some populations. Concepts like "Only a fat baby is a healthy baby" and "Eat, don't talk" still exist. Many major joyous holidays are associated with eating and overeating. Think of Thanksgiving dinners, Passover seders, and even Halloween (trick or treat means candy, candy, candy). For the lower socioeconomic groups, high-calorie foods, particularly starches, are cheaper than proteins, and diets tend to be excessively high in foods that help put on extra weight.

What can we conclude? Obesity and morbid obesity are complex problems and there appear to be numerous related and unrelated factors involved.

NOTES

1. S. C. Wooley, O. W. Wooley, and S. Dyrenforth, "The Case Against Radical Intervention," *American Journal of Clinical Nutrition* 33 (1980): 465–71.

2. J. H. Payne, "Obesity," *Annals of Surgery* 120 (1970): 513.

3. E. J. Drenick, "Definition and Health Consequences of Morbid Obesity," *Surgical Clinics of North America* 59 (1979): 963–76.

4. Ibid.

5. Bray et al., "The Control of Food Intake: Effects of Dieting and Intestinal Bypass," *Surgical Clinics of North America* 59 (1979): 1043–54.

6. Drenick, "Definition and Health Consequences of Morbid Obesity."

7. A. J. Stunkard, T. T. Foch, and Z. Hrubec, "A Twin Study of Human Obesity," *JAMA* 256 (1986): 51–54.

8. L. A. Scuro and O. Bosello, "The Problem of Classifying Obesity," *World Journal of Surgery* 5 (1981): 789–94.

9. Stunkard, Foch, and Hrubec, "A Twin Study of Human Obesity."

10. Scuro and Bosello, "The Problem of Classifying Obesity."

11. J. Friedman in G. Kolata, "Researchers Find Hormone Causes a Loss of Weight," *New York Times*, July 27, 1955.

12. N. Wade, "Genetic Cause Found for Some Cases in Human Obesity," *New York Times*, June 24, 1997.

13. K. A. Halmi et al., "Psychiatric Diagnosis of Morbidly Obese Gastric Bypass Patients," *American Journal of Psychiatry* 137 (1980): 470–72.

14. K. Gentry, J. D. Halverson, and S. Heisler, "Psychologic Assessment of Morbid Obese Patients Undergoing Gastric Bypass: A Comparison of Preoperative and Postoperative Adjustment," *Surgery* 95 (1984): 215–20.

15. A. H. Crisp and B. McGuiness, "Jolly Fat: Relation between Obesity and Psychoneurosis in General Population," *British Medical Journal* 1 (1976): 7–9.

16. E. S. Parham, H. C. Keng, and I. Mohiuddin, "Sensitivity to Psychological Hunger Cues: Are the Obese Really Different?" *Nutrition Reports International* 12 (1975): 383–86.

17. P. J. Lanzisera et al., "Minnesota Mutiphasic Profiles of the Morbidly Obese," *Henry Ford Hospital Medical Journal* 36 (1988): 78–81.

18. Gentry, Halverson, and Heisler, "Psychologic Assessment of Morbid Obese Patients Undergoing Gastric Bypass."

6

What Does the Term "Morbid" Mean?

Let us eat and drink; for tomorrow we shall die.
　　　　　　　　　　　　　　　　—Ecclesiastes (Bible)

Now it's time to justify the word "morbid" in the term "morbid obesity."
As you'll recall, *morbid obesity* has been defined as a weight level that is
at least 100 pounds over one's ideal weight, which is likely to bring about
major medical or physical problems relating to the obesity. What major
medical and physical problems are we talking about?

DEATH

The most serious problem is death: the heavier one is, the shorter one's
life span. This is especially disastrous for very heavy individuals, those I
call superobese. In one recent study of a group of sixteen superobese
patients, all weighing over 650 pounds, only two lived beyond thirty-nine
years of age. Occasionally we hear about or see on television some unfortunate individual who attracts public attention because of his or her massive size. It's usually something like the doorway is being enlarged so he
can get out of the house, or he is given a motorcycle to get around because
he is unable to support himself on his own legs, or some new highly pub-
licized diet is being tried. Then it all ends, usually abruptly, with death at
an early age.

　　Several years ago I was asked to see a very obese patient who was in the hospital because of terrible skin ulcers on his legs. The ulcers were directly related to his weight, which was over 400 pounds, and to the poor blood circulation occurring in heavy people. Everyone agreed that he needed to lose a considerable amount of weight if these ulcers were to heal. I talked to the man about gastric bypass operation, and although he was interested, he thought he would try dieting one more time. This sounded reasonable. He was discharged from the hospital with instructions to call me if he changed his mind about an operation. After about four years, I received a telephone call from the director of the nursing home where this patient was living. I was told that he had gained more weight, and his legs would no longer support him. He was literally living on the floor. His skin color had a greyish appearance and he did not look at all well. I told the nursing home director to get the patient into an ambulance and get him to our Emergency Room as soon as possible. In the meantime, I contacted several of my internal-medicine colleagues to help me evaluate and correct his medical problems so that he could be operated on. Four more days passed without seeing the patient. Then I received another call from the nursing home director. "I guess I should tell you what happened," he said. "The ambulance came, and as four of us were lifting him on to a stretcher, he suddenly gasped and died." Make no mistake about it, morbid obesity is potentially a lethal condition!

Death can occur suddenly without warning in morbidly obese people, even if they are not in the over-400-pound superobese category. The sudden death syndrome sometimes affects these patients. Those who have the syndrome will suddenly die without any warning. Some experts believe it is due to an irregularity of the function of the heart. Fortunately it is not common, but I have seen it in my practice. One of my patients who was scheduled for surgery never showed up at the hospital. Some time later I found out that she had succumbed to this sudden death syndrome several days before her scheduled admission date.

This sudden death syndrome can occur in nonobese people also, but is about forty times more common in the morbidly obese population. There was one study by Drenick and Fisher[1] describing sixty such deaths in morbidly obese patients. Eight occurred in patients waiting for obesity surgery, like my patient, twenty-two in patients within ten days after the operation, and thirty were late postoperative deaths, occurring more than four weeks after surgery. These last thirty patients were still very obese.

Finally I should cite a very important study from a Veterans Administration hospital in California which was reported in 1980. Dr. Ernst

Drenick studied a group of two hundred morbidly obese men, aged twenty-three to seventy years who had an average weight of about 315 pounds. After an average follow-up period of about seven and a half years, he found that fifty of them, or 25 percent, had died. Most deaths were due to diseases of the heart and circulatory systems even in the younger patients. Two choked on food during eating sprees, and many died from accidents, including drowning, gunshot wounds, automobile accidents, and drug overdoses. But the major point was this. These death rates were compared to death rates in normal-sized males in the general population. There were twelve times as many deaths in the youngest morbidly obese group, those from twenty-five to thirty-four years of age, than would be expected in normal-sized males of similar ages. In the thirty-five- to forty-four-year-olds, death rates were six times greater, and in the older morbidly obese patients, death was two to three times greater. Morbid obesity is obviously a potentially lethal condition, according to Drenick[2] and me.

All of this sounds very dismal, and it is. Our goal in medicine and for those of us who specialize in surgical treatment is to prevent these deaths, and also to try to improve the various medical problems that could lead to an early death. We also hope to improve the physical disabilities that make life a burden for many morbidly obese patients.

The list of these medical and physical problems is a long one, and there have been many studies, including those by Drenick,[3] Rimm et al.,[4] Austin et al.,[5] Printen et al.,[6] Imam and Sowers,[7] and Sims and Berchtold,[8] on the association of these problems with the obese population. One such study by Rimm et al. involved questionnaires that were answered by over 70,000 women who experienced varying degrees of obesity. In one part of the study the authors compared the incidence of certain medical problems in the heaviest group, those averaging 85 percent over ideal weight (which included morbidly obese women) with the least heavy group, those only 10 percent overweight. Certain of these medical conditions were found to be significantly more common in the most obese group. These were: diabetes, 4.5 times more common; high blood pressure, over 3 times; gallbladder disease, 2.5 times; gout, 2.5 times; underactive thyroid function, 1.5 times; other thyroid gland problems, 1.5 times; heart disease, 1.5 times; arthritis, 1.5 times; and jaundice, almost 1.5 times more common. Since this 85 percent overweight group included many women who were not quite heavy enough to be considered morbidly obese, the actual incidence of these conditions in the morbidly obese group is probably even worse.

DIABETES MELLITUS

Diabetes is a particularly interesting problem in these patients. The association of diabetes with obesity, even slight obesity, has been known for many years. In morbid obesity, diabetes may be three to five times more prevalent than in normal-sized patients. Possibly 25 to 50 percent of all morbidly obese patients may have either true diabetes or chemical changes in the body suggestive of a prediabetic condition. There does appear to be an increased tendency to develop diabetes as these patients get older and heavier. In some cases it seems to take twenty to twenty-five years of morbid obesity to finally develop the diabetes. Some authorities claim that diabetes in most morbidly obese patients is relatively mild, and that death and serious complications of the disease are uncommon. But many of the patients need daily insulin injections for control, and sometimes large doses are required. Of even more importance is the fact that diabetes in these patients seems to act as a "cofactor" with other medical problems responsible for cardiac and circulatory deaths. Some authorities think that the most dangerous situation in regard to diabetes occurs when patients rapidly regain weight lost after dieting.

I find it very interesting that these diabetic morbidly obese people actually produce an increased amount of insulin. The problem appears to be that the body's sensitivity to insulin is decreased and that a resistance to insulin has developed.

HIGH BLOOD PRESSURE

High blood pressure (hypertension) is another major problem that may be associated with morbid obesity. It is about three times more common in these patients, but the problem is even worse in the younger morbidly obese individuals. In patients aged twenty to forty-four years, high blood pressure is five times more prevalent in those who are morbidly obese. Some say that the situation is even worse in obese men than women. I read one report that said for each additional 10 kilograms (22 pounds) in weight, blood pressure goes up about two to three millimeters. High blood pressure is another one of those cofactors leading to serious cardiac and circulatory problems.

HEART DISEASE AND STROKES

Heart disease and strokes are increased in morbid obesity, and are probably related to the cofactors mentioned above, and also to high blood cholesterol levels. Another probable factor is the limitation of physical activity and exercise in these patients because of their excessive weight. Angina (severe chest pain), myocardial infarcts (heart attacks), and sudden death syndrome occur with greater frequency. These problems often occur in a younger age group, such as those under forty years as well as in elderly patients, and the heart attacks are often fatal.

ARTHRITIS

Arthritis and other ailments of the muscles, bones, and joints are among the most common physical problems causing disability and pain in the morbidly obese population. The back and weight-bearing joints, such as hips, knees, and ankles, are especially affected. The degree of disability ranges from relatively minor to totally crippling. Many patients are restricted to the use of walkers or even wheelchairs. The saddest part is that corrective joint replacement would relieve many of the symptoms, but such surgery cannot be done because of the massive weight of the patients and the increased anesthetic risk and risk of infection. A high failure rate of these operations would occur, not only because the operations would be difficult technically, but also because the new joints would deteriorate rapidly due to the stress put on them by the body's massive weight. Some of these patients are relatively young and their limitation of activity is pitiful to see. This, of course, means no exercise programs, and without exercise weight only tends to increase further.

GALLSTONES

Another medical problem that we see very frequently is gallbladder disease and gallstones. The reason for increased gallbladder disease is not completely understood, but may be related to an increase in the secretion of cholesterol by the liver into the bile, forming cholesterol gallstones. This is three to four times more common in the morbidly obese. About 35 percent of these people have either had their gallbladders removed before seeking surgical aid for obesity, or need the gallbladder removed at the time of their obesity operation. Like some of the above problems, the situation gets worse with increasing age, and also with greater weight.

Serum Lipids

There is a tendency for the morbidly obese to have elevated levels of cholesterol, although many patients have surprisingly normal levels (cholesterol should be below 200 mc/dl). The same is true with triglycerides, fatty substances in the blood. But some do have extraordinarily high levels.

Respiratory Problems

One final and very common problem relates to the respiratory system and the lungs. Most morbidly obese patients become short of breath with relatively little physical activity. This breathlessness may further limit their activity. Climbing stairs, for example, becomes an impossibility. Some patients are severely limited, and some even need an oxygen tank nearby at all times. Asthma seems to be common.

When measurements are made of the oxygen in their bloodstream, the morbidly obese are generally well below normal. The function of their lungs ranges from relatively normal to absolutely disastrous. Their diaphragms are usually pushed up by the increased abdominal mass and intra-abdominal pressures, resulting in a decrease in lung volume and a reduced capacity to breath deeply. The muscles of the chest are inefficient and expansion of the lungs becomes more difficult. The worst lung problem that we see is the Pickwickian syndrome, also called Obesity Hypoventilation syndrome or Obesity Sleep Apnea. This is extremely fascinating from a medical perspective, but it is very serious. I'll discuss this in greater detail later, but it includes such problems as falling asleep at inappropriate times, retaining high levels of carbon dioxide in the body, and eventually acute respiratory distress, heart problems, and sometimes death.

OTHER PROBLEMS

There are plenty of other problems associated with morbid obesity. For example, certain types of cancers have been shown to be more prevalent in these patients. In men, cancers of the large intestine, the rectum, and the prostate gland are more common. In women, increased incidence of cancers of the gallbladder, the bile passages, ovaries, breasts, and uterus have been reported. Cancers of the uterus are somewhere between five to almost twenty times more common, and the survival after treatment is decreased.

Problems with the circulation of the legs are often seen, ranging from terrible ulcerations of the skin, to an increased incidence of inflammation and blood clots in the leg veins. This may result in blood clots traveling to the lungs (pulmonary emboli) and death.

Hernias (protrusion of internal body structure through the abdominal wall) are common, especially hernias around the navel. This is probably because of the marked increase in pressure within the abdomen in morbidly obese patients, which weakens the abdominal wall muscles. Other medical problems reported in these patients include inflammation of the pancreas, kidney disease, menstrual disorders, infertility, dermatoses, cataracts of the eye, increased infections (due to poor circulation), psychiatric disorders, suicides, and drug overdoses.

PREGNANCY

Pregnancy, when it occurs in morbidly obese women, may have more complications, including toxemia, high blood pressure, and diabetes. Miscarriages are twice as common, pregnancies may last longer, babies may be heavier, birth defects are more common, and Caesarean sections are necessary more often. Infant mortality is supposed to be about two and a half times greater with morbidly obese mothers.

Finally, there are all sorts of social and economic troubles, but these will be discussed later.

This is the chapter that the health insurance companies should be sure to read. Some of them still think that these operations are purely for cosmetic purposes, rather than for treatment of a serious medical condition.

Sure, many of the patients look better after losing a lot of weight, but we are talking about serious health problems that accompany the obesity.

NOTES

1. E. J. Drenick and J. S. Fisler, "Sudden Cardiac Arrest in Morbidly Obese Surgical Patients Unexplained after Autopsy," *American Journal of Surgery* 155 (1988): 720–26.

2. E. J. Drenick, "Definition and Health Consequences of Morbid Obesity," *Surgical Clinics of North America* 59 (1979): 963–75.

3. Ibid.

4. A. A. Rimm et al., "Relationship of Obesity and Disease in 73,532 Weight-Conscious Women," *Public Health Reports* 90 (1975): 44–51.

5. H. Austin et al., "Endometrial Cancer, Obesity, and Body Fat Distribution," *Cancer Research* 51 (1991): 568–72.

6. K. J. Printen et al., "Venous Thromboembolism in the Morbidly Obese," *Surgery, Gynecology & Obstetrics* 147 (1978): 63–64.

7. K. Imam and J. R. Sowers, "Obesity and Hypertension: A Review," *Henry Ford Hospital Medical Journal* 36 (1988): 82–87.

8. E. A. H. Sims and P. Berchtold, "Obesity and Hypertension," *JAMA* 247 (1982): 49–52.

7

A Short History: Intestinal Bypass

They are as sick that surfeit with too much, as that starve with nothing.
—Shakespeare, *The Merchant of Venice*

Surgeons have been involved with the care of very obese patients for many years. At first, our task was to treat some of the complications of obesity. Neurosurgeons and orthopedic surgeons have treated the various back problems that plague the very obese, and orthopedists have repaired and, more recently, replaced diseased joints in the legs of these unfortunate patients. Cardiac surgeons have been operating on the hearts of obese and other patients for about forty years. Vascular surgeons have treated the leg ulcers of these patients, and there were even some operations devised and performed in the 1950s for the management of high blood pressure. All of these treated the effects of obesity, not the obesity itself.

The actual beginnings of the surgical attack on obesity may have occurred in Sweden, but it's been difficult to get complete information about this. According to Dr. Philip Sandblom of Lund, Sweden, a Swedish surgeon named Henrickson from Gothenburg tried to control his patient's weight by removing part of the small intestine. Apparently the patient lost a lot of weight, but nutritional problems resulted. The exact date of this operation is somewhat uncertain. This bit of history was mentioned, in 1980, in a book about the surgical management of obesity by Dr. E. E. Mason,[1] himself a pioneer in this field.

The real, meaningful beginnings of surgical intervention occurred in Minneapolis at the University of Minnesota. Drs. Arnold Kremen and

John Linner were studying the absorption of nitrogen in the small intestine after eliminating either the *jejunum* (upper small intestine) or the *ileum* (lower small intestine). There had been a great deal of interest in the nutritional effects of removing parts of the small intestine. Many patients, through the years, had had large portions of the small intestine removed because of cancer or other diseases of the intestine. Most of these patients were not obese. When more than half of their small intestine was removed, reduced absorption of nutrients was seen. If 75 percent or more of the intestine was removed, weight loss occurred, but serious nutritional difficulties often resulted, including deficiencies of potassium, magnesium, calcium, and protein. It was gradually learned that those who could endure the weight loss, such as morbidly obese patients, could better tolerate the removal of much of their intestinal tract.

Kremen and Linner wrote a scientific paper in 1954 discussing their experimental animal studies, and also described an operation they performed on a very obese woman. This thirty-four-year-old woman had weighed 385 pounds but reduced this to 275 pounds by very strict dieting. In an operation on April 9, 1954, these surgeons bypassed much of her small intestine, leaving her with 36 inches of the jejunum and 18 inches of the ileum to digest and absorb her food. This left her with only about 25 percent of her functioning small intestine. Actually, over the years we have learned that leaving her with 25 percent was not radical enough for a good weight loss in a morbidly obese patient. But her weight did come down to 240 pounds. Eventually, in 1971 she underwent surgery again, and her bypass was shortened to 16 inches of jejunum and 6 inches of ileum. Her weight then dropped to a low of 171 pounds and eventually leveled off at 190 pounds. Eight years later, she died of a heart attack at the age of sixty. She was the first well-documented patient to have an operation directed specifically against obesity, the jejunoileal bypass, also called the *intestinal bypass*.

Dr. Edward Mason, a major pioneer in this field of surgery, who was also a University of Minnesota trained surgeon, performed two similar operations in 1954. His second operation was a *jejunocolic bypass*, where the entire ileum was bypassed. In this operation, the functioning part of the jejunum was connected to the large intestine (colon). This patient apparently had a lot of diarrhea and required some additional surgery. We will hear much more about Dr. Mason in later chapters.

Dr. Howard Payne, in California, then started an active program in 1956 for the treatment of morbidly obese patients using intestinal bypass surgery. His first operations were very radical jejunocolic procedures,

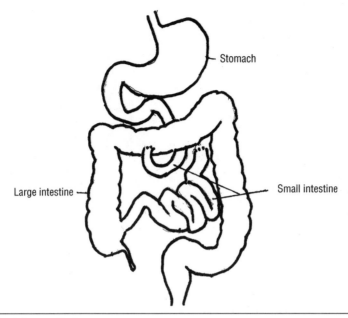

Fig. 4. Jejunocolic bypass

where he bypassed all but the first 15 inches of jejunum, which he then connected to the midportion of the colon (Fig. 4). So he actually bypassed about half of the colon also. A very major weight loss occurred, but the complications were overwhelming. These included severe diarrhea, deficiencies of certain "electrolytes" such as potassium and calcium, and liver failure. His original plan was to reoperate on these patients, adding intestinal length to improve absorption of calories and electrolytes when the patient had lost the desired weight. When Payne and others evaluated the results of these jejunocolic operations, it was agreed by all that this was not a good operation because of variable weight loss and severe nutritional problems, and that it should no longer be performed.

But the fact that a significant weight loss could sometimes occur with these operations was encouraging. The key thing appeared to be establishing a balance between poor absorption of calories and an acceptable amount of absorption of the necessary nutrients, including protein, potassium, calcium, and magnesium. The jejunoileal bypass, retaining part of the jejunum and also part of the ileum, became the favored operation in the 1960s and into the 1970s.

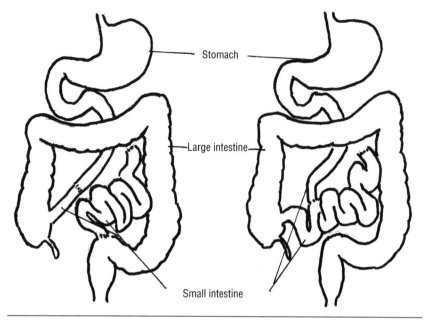

Fig. 5. End-to-end and end-to-side intestinal bypasses

VARIATIONS IN THE JEJUNO-ILEAL BYPASSES

But the big question was how much of the jejunum and how much of the ileum should be kept and how much should be bypassed? Should the functioning part of the jejunum be connected to the end of the functioning part of the ileum (end-to-end operation) or to the side of the functioning ileum (end-to-side operation) (Fig. 5)? The theoretic disadvantage of the end-to-side operation was that food leaving the functioning jejunum could enter the ileum and back up into the bypassed or nonfunctioning ileum with the result that additional calories could be absorbed. Strangely enough, this point was never totally answered. Not everyone believed this, but I did, and I used the end-to-end operation.

Every surgeon had his own idea as to how much functional jejunum and ileum should be left. Payne advocated 14 inches of jejunum and 4 inches of ileum. William Scott from Vanderbilt University first used 12 inches and 12 inches, but changed this to 12 inches of jejunum and 6 inches of ileum. Peter Salmon, a Minnesota-trained Canadian surgeon, used 10 inches of jejunum and 20 inches of ileum. Finally, Henry Buchwald from Minnesota connected 16 inches of jejunum to 1.6 inches of ileum. While possible advantages and disadvantages were discussed far and wide, it really seemed that the resulting weight losses from these various procedures were all fairly similar. It seemed that the total length of functioning small intestine should probably not have been much more than 20 inches, nor much less than 18 inches.

I used 12 inches of jejunum and 8 inches of ileum, a reasonable compromise I thought. I frequently measured the length of the entire small intestine in my patients at the time of the operation and found that it averaged 200 inches. So I was bypassing 90 percent of the small intestine in my operations. Since some patients had a slightly longer intestinal length and some a shorter length, the actual percentage of bypass varied from about 87 to 93 percent. This did not seem to matter in terms of resulting weight loss.

Well, the jejunoileal or intestinal bypass caught on, and was the treatment of choice for morbidly obese patients who were unable to lose weight by dieting. Possibly, in excess of 100,000 of these operations were done in the United States during the 1960s and 1970s. However, a new, completely different operation, the gastric bypass, was being developed during this period, and this new operation would eventually make the intestinal bypass obsolete. More about this in chapter 15.

NOTE

1. E. E. Mason, *Surgical Treatment of Obesity* (Philadelphia: W. B. Saunders, 1981).

8

My First Operations

The beginning is the most important part of the work.
—Plato, *The Republic*

As I mentioned earlier, my interest in operating on morbidly obese patients began when I was in Kansas City, in 1971. I only did a few of these operations during this time, possibly because I still was unsure that the patient would benefit from the operations. Was I really going to help these people by this operation? I think it's a good thing for a doctor, particularly a surgeon, to have a lot of questions about what he or she does.

My first patient was Roger, the 340-pound man I mentioned in chapter 1. Then I operated on a woman in the mid-200-pound range. This didn't seem so hard. But the next patient was middle-aged and over 400 pounds. And the patient after that weighed over 500 pounds. But the strange thing was that the operation on the 400-pound woman wasn't all that difficult. It seemed that because of all the fat in the abdomen, everything was pushed upward toward the surface. I don't mean to imply that these are easy operations. They are not. They are major operations in every respect. But the point is that it doesn't necessarily get harder just because one patient is bigger than the next.

Operating on 500-plus-pound patients is hard. One woman was the biggest patient I had ever seen, let alone operated on. All of these operations are very physical procedures. The surgeons are constantly pulling and pushing the heavy, thick abdominal wall and the large deposits of fat within the abdomen in order to expose the organs that are being cut and sewn. The instruments are the same as we use on nonobese patients. It can be hard physical labor for the surgeon. I always explain to my surgical residents, "These are weight reduction operations; I lose 2 or 3 pounds with every operation!"

People often ask me how I can cut through so much fat. Actually, cutting through the fat is the easiest part. Retracting it and keeping it out of the way can be difficult, and gaining exposure to all of the organs involved in the operation can be a problem. Other aspects of the management of these patients can be very difficult. Starting an intravenous line, or drawing blood from a vein is often hard because the veins are buried deep beneath the skin and its underlying fatty layer. Measuring blood pressure is sometimes inaccurate because the cuff of the blood pressure meter may not be large enough to fit around the arm correctly.

ORDINARY HOSPITAL PROBLEMS

Even the simple comforts that every patient in the hospital should have may be lacking for these morbidly obese patients. A hospital gown? It is often not big enough for the 400- and 500-pound patients. Sometimes two gowns are sewn together in order to cover the patient. The hospital bed and the chair in the room may not be large enough. One hospital I've worked in had their carpenters build a large platform bed and a settee for the biggest of the patients.

Weighing the patient before the operation is very important. We have to know at what weight we started so that we can eventually calculate the amount of weight lost from the operation. But weighing the patient can be a real problem. Most scales only go up to 350 pounds. I always emphasize vigorously to the residents and nurses the importance of getting an accurate preoperative weight. (Nothing gets me madder than not having an accurate preoperative weight. How can I know how much weight the patient is losing without it!) So, through the years they have been very innovative. Sometimes the patients were weighed on 2 scales, one foot on one and the other foot on the second scale. Surprisingly, this sometimes works. At other times, patients are taken down to the basement of the hospital where the meat scales are located. This is terrible! Think how embarrassing this must be for the poor patients. Fortunately, in more recent years electronic scales have become available. I don't know how high they go, but all my patients have been able to be weighed on the electronic scales.

Other problems include transportation: getting patients to the X-ray Department or to the operating room or anywhere. If it's a long distance, they can't walk, and some are so disabled that they can't even walk a short distance. So, put them in a wheelchair. Ordinary wheelchairs may not be large enough, although there are extra-large wheelchairs available in some hospitals. Maybe a litter could be used. Again, it may not be large enough, and there may be problems just getting the patient on the litter. Sometimes the patients are transported from one part of the hospital to another on their own hospital bed, but the beds are heavy and the patients are heavy as well, and it may take two or more hospital orderlies to move the bed. This can be very embarrassing for the patient. I had one very sensitive patient who asked me how we were going to transport her to the X-ray Department. I asked her, in return, how she wanted to go. She answered, "Not by wheelchair. They'll stuff me in it with difficulty, and then pull me out of it when we get to X-ray, and everyone will have a good laugh at my expense!" She was absolutely right to be upset about this. Her life was hard enough without extra ridicule. (We sent her down in her own bed.)

Getting the patient off the bed and onto the X-ray table or onto the operating room table is also a major problem at times. This transferral is especially hard when the patient is somewhat disabled or extra heavy. The hospital in Kansas City had just bought a new machine that was used for transferring patients from one surface to another, such as from a bed to an X-ray table. It worked by sliding a metal panel under the patient, and then moving away from the first surface it delivered the patient to the second surface. When my 500-pound patient was put on this machine, it broke under the weight of the patient.

In the operating room there are problems, other than the operation itself, due to the sheer bulk of some of the patients. The anesthesiologists often have a hard time putting in the endotracheal tube before the operation begins. The endotracheal tube is a short, rigid plastic tube that is put in through the mouth down into the trachea, or windpipe. It is used for giving the gas anesthesia for the operation, and also for giving the patient air and oxygen to breath. It is vitally important. But many of the patients have short, fat inflexible necks, or virtually no necks at all, and getting this tube into the right place can be a nightmare for the anesthesiologists. If they put the patient asleep first, and then have difficulty getting the tube into the trachea, the patient could possibly die from lack of oxygen. The anesthesiologists must therefore assess the situation before starting, and if they anticipate that there may be difficulties, they may put in the tube while the patient is awake ("awake intubation"). It is safe and effective, but may be uncomfortable for the patient although a spray and gargle with a local anesthetic is used to numb the throat.

Another problem in the operating room involves putting in the urinary catheter, particularly in females. I won't go into details on this, but the legs are often heavy and fat. Spreading them far enough to expose the genital area, and spreading the labia enough to find the urinary outlet can be incredibly difficult.

After the operation, lifting the still asleep patient back to the bed or litter is another significant task. Somehow it always seems that the smallest nurses do most of the lifting.

There are many other problems in the postoperative period. One problem that first occurred in Kansas City was when we needed an accurate X-ray of the abdomen in one of the very heavy patients. We couldn't get it. X-rays just cannot penetrate through the entire abdomen in a very obese patient. All we got was a very hazy image that was of no value. Very valuable diagnostic procedures are therefore not available for all of these patients. I later learned that the soft tissue X-ray technique of CAT scanning may also be unavailable for these patients. One of the problems with this technique is that the patients may be too large to fit into the tunnel where the CAT scans are conducted.

My early experiences with the morbidly obese in Kansas City were important opportunities to learn. I began to learn who the morbidly obese are, what the operations are like, and what the problems and benefits of the procedures are.

Managing these morbidly obese patients, as you have seen, is not easy. This is particularly true with those that are 300, 400, or 500 pounds in weight. However, in later chapters, you will see that the alternatives are not so good, and that even the difficulties with these patients in surgery are worthwhile.

9

But What About Dieting?

A man must take fat with the lean.
—Charles Dickens, *David Copperfield*

In reading through the previous chapters I may have given the impression that the only treatment for severe obesity is surgical. This is certainly not true, although as you will see, the overwhelming majority of morbidly obese patients do appear to respond better to surgery than to other available types of treatment. I think we should spend time here reviewing the types of treatments that are not surgical.

I have a very positive feeling about diets and their role in treating obesity. Diets are the baseline, the foundation, the beginning of all attacks against obesity. All obese patients, including the morbidly obese, must start with weight-reduction diets. The successful patients are the fortunate ones. As difficult as dieting is, and it is difficult, everything else, including surgery, is even more so. We doctors only wish that dietary therapy was more successful than it is.

A Brief History of Diets

Rigid, formal, "scientific" dieting is a relatively new phenomenon, mostly of the nineteenth and twentieth centuries. Earlier than that, most people either weren't interested, didn't need it, or couldn't afford to be bothered. While there certainly were overweight people in the distant past, and probably some of them made an effort to control their weight, not much was written about it. There are no weight-reduction diet books from ancient Rome or even the Middle Ages, at least as far as I know. Life span was shorter than it is now, and there was probably little concern about a shortened length of life due to excessive weight. I'm sure there was more concern about the periodic plagues and natural disasters than there was about obesity.

Let me present a brief account of some of the more notable dietary programs in the past. One of the earliest accounts of successful weight loss with dieting involved an Italian, Luigi Cornaro, who lived in the sixteenth century. Cornaro was obese and suffered from gout and stomach problems. At age forty, he put himself on a rigid diet of only 12 ounces of food and 14 ounces of liquids each day. His health improved remarkably with his loss of weight and he lived to a fine old age of ninety-one. Of course, he wrote a book about his experiences, *A Treatise of the Benefits of a Sober Life*, in 1558. This was one of the first diet books based on the personal experiences of the author.

The next notable dieter was Dr. George Cheyne, who was born in Scotland in 1673. Cheyne was also very obese and suffered from some of the problems that we still see in our obese patients, shortness of breath and easy fatigability. Weight loss did not come easy to him. He tried a variety of medicines, induced vomiting, and then used opium and calomel (a strong cathartic used to bring about bowel evacuation), and only felt worse. Next came the spas of Bath and Bristol. He then heard about and tried a milk diet, and lost much weight. But his story isn't over yet. Cheyne acquired pains in his stomach, which he treated with vigorous exercise and purgatives. Chewing quinine seemed to help, but he again developed a hearty appetite. His weight rose and rose, until he was almost 450 pounds. (The story sounds familiar, doesn't it?) He complained of asthma, sores, and infections. Finally, he achieved success with a vegetarian diet coupled with milk, tea, and coffee. The weight came off and his diseases vanished. Of course he wrote a book, or several of them. One of his books was entitled *The English Malady*, referring to the weight of the body and the weight of the soul.

Cheyne's writings were widely quoted in Britain and also in the British colonies in the New World. But Americans in the early 1800s tended to be lean, not fat. Leanness was the national image. American soldiers in 1850 weighed 147 pounds and were 5 feet, 7 inches tall. However, by the mid-1800s we start to hear more about diets and weight reduction.

Sylvester Graham was an itinerant lecturer, originally on the temperance circuit, but expanded his targets to masturbation, cholera, and finally gluttony. He wrote and lectured extensively on what he considered to be healthy eating and a "natural" weight. A controversial figure, he would have thrived these days on TV talk shows and on the best-seller list. His dietary program was a simple one, with emphasis on vegetables, fruits, wheat bread, rice, and pure water. Those who read his work were supposed to eat slowly and chew their food well. To be avoided were all spices, condiments, gravies, tea, coffee, tobacco, butter, and pastries. His critics pictured the Grahamites as dried-up human skeletons and Graham was called Dr. Sawdust. But his message persisted, and he had a lasting influence on generations of health-conscious dieters.

Unlike Graham who was thin or even gaunt, William Banting was overweight. In fact, he weighed more than 200 pounds. He lived in London, worked as an undertaker, and slowly watched his weight rise. He tried the usual combinations of treatment, exercise (it only increased his appetite), spas, purgatives and diuretics to reduce body water, and Turkish baths. All failed. Finally on the advice of his doctor he tried dieting. His diet consisted mainly of lean meat, dry toast, soft-boiled eggs, and green vegetables. His diet consisted of 21 to 27 ounces of solid food and 30 ounces of liquid per day. It worked. He lost more than 50 pounds and felt himself a new man. His *Letter on Corpulence Addressed to the Public* in the 1860s sold more than 50,000 copies. His influence was felt even in America. The term "banting" was used for describing this now popular method of dieting, with its emphasis on lean meats and low levels of fat.

The interest in weight loss continued, and so did the weight of Americans, as we began to approach the twentieth century according to Schwartz.[1] There were several new developments, however. Horace Fletcher, an overweight American, experimented not on diets, but on new ways of eating. He developed Fletcherism, a doctrine that advocated slow, careful chewing of all foods. Even milk and soups had to be chewed. Most foods required about thirty seconds of chewing per mouthful, but high-fiber foods might need several minutes. Fletcher's dinners might take 2,500 chews over a thirty-minute period. Eat-Your-Food-Slowly Societies were proposed. Fletcher wrote and lectured extensively, and slow chewing of less food became widely popular. Many of our current popular dietary programs still suggest chewing all food slowly and carefully.

Finally, there began to be dietary programs combined with other possible methods for producing weight loss, such as exercise programs, mas-

sage treatments, use of skin preparations, electrotherapy (electrical stimulation of muscle groups), and all sorts of combinations of drugs. For
example, Marjorie Hamilton's Quadruple Combination System of Fat
Reduction—a modified banting diet combined with enemas to decrease
calorie absorption, juice of half a lemon twice a day, Indian club exer-
cises, mineral waters, and Healthstone Obesity Powder (sodium carbonate, Epsom salts, Glauber salts, and saltpeter).

PRINCIPLES

Let's move away from history and on to the present, the second half of
the twentieth century. The basic principles of acceptable diets are:

1. They must provide less than the patient's energy requirements.
2. They must provide all nutrient requirements.
3. They must be acceptable to the patient.
4. They must be sustained long-term.
5. They must not impair health.
6. Effectiveness will depend on the foods not eaten.

Monotonous diets will not work long-term. Crash diets are difficult
to stay on, and compensatory overeating may follow. Also, very rapid
major weight losses may burn off lean body tissue, including muscle,
rather than fat. Weight loss during the first and second weeks may be
mostly water loss. Very impressive, but easily regained. Diets not provid-
ing all nutrient requirements may be dangerous, injuring health and even
causing death.

Other principles in most diets include eating several meals per day, not
just one big meal, having regular set mealtimes, eating and chewing slowly,
and stopping when full. Snacking is prohibited. Expensive and complicated
diets are best avoided. Dieters should shop for food *after* eating.

There is no shortage of printed material about dieting and weight loss.
For example, books in the 1970s included *Calories Don't Count*; *The
Doctor's Quick Weight Loss Diet*; *Slim Chances in a Fat World*; *Act Thin,
Stay Thin*; *Eating Is Okay*; *Take It Off and Keep It Off*; *Live Longer Now*;
The Fat Counter Guide; *The Doctor's Metabolic Diet*; *The Last Chance
Diet*; and *Fasting Is a Way of Life*. Two more recent books were *The Car-
bohydrate Addict's Diet* and *The T-Factor Fat Gram Counter*.

So, there are many diets and many types of diets. This correctly implies that there is no such thing as a perfect diet that always works well under all circumstances. Americans spend more than 3 billion dollars on commercial diets. Since this book is not a "diet book," I will try only to summarize the different types of diets, including conventional diets, starvation and very-low-calorie diets, self-help and commercial dietary programs, and behavioral modification.

CONVENTIONAL DIETS

Conventional dietary therapy involves the use of low, but not drastically low-calorie intake with some balance of nutrients, vitamins, and minerals. Caloric intake may be in the range of 1,200 to 2,000 calories per day. Some of these diets emphasize certain types of foods to the exclusion of other foods, and some have their own particular gimmicks to help in the process of weight loss. The Stillman diet involves a high water intake, eight glasses per day, in addition to lean meat, fish, low-fat cheeses, poultry, and eggs. The Pritikin diet is very low in fat, carbohydrate, and salt, with emphasis on fruit, vegetables, breads, and cereals. The "Calories Don't Count" diet is high in fat and protein, and includes one-third of a cup of vegetable oil per day. The Peterkin diet emphasizes bread, cereals, fruit, and vegetables, with low meat and milk intake. The "Anti-Stress" diet is a balanced diet, but suggests dieting only three days per week. Most of these diets have resulted in weight loss, but the amount lost is not satisfactory enough for the heaviest patients, those who are morbidly obese. Very few individuals have enough patience and "staying power" to continue on these diets for a long-term period. This is particularly true of the morbidly obese group.[2]

VERY-LOW-CALORIE DIETS

If cutting down calories to a moderate extent resulted in some weight loss, why not cut calories to a very low level to get an even greater weight loss? This is a logical question discussed by Van Itallie and Kral,[3] Drenick,[4] Wadden et al.,[5] and Bernstein and Van Itallie,[6] and it brought about the concept of very-low-calorie or starvation diets. These included the liquid-protein diets of the 1970s, the "Cambridge" diet of the 1980s and the more recent well-publicized very-low-calorie diets, such as Optifast, Medifast, and Health Management Resources. Very-low-calorie diets provide about 400 to 800 calories per day. Most include a high-quality protein component, attempting to preserve lean muscle mass while the patient loses weight. Some of these programs have involved lengthy hospitalizations while the patient is under direct medical supervision. In some of the newer and popular programs the diet includes a powder containing proteins from milk or egg sources. This is mixed with water and taken three to five times a day. In other diets, the protein comes from food such as lean meat, fish, or poultry. Vitamin and mineral supplements are included, and large quantities of noncaloric liquids are required.

These very-low-calorie diets are potentially dangerous. They are not suggested for patients with histories of heart problems, or blood vessel, kidney, or liver disease. Medical supervision with frequent examinations and laboratory studies are often recommended. There were fifty-eight deaths reported by Van Itallie and Kral,[7] Drenick,[8] and Bernstein and Van Itallie[9] in patients on liquid-protein diets, and six deaths in people on the Cambridge diet noted by Wadden and associates.[10] The newer programs are apparently much safer. With these drastic programs one would expect some complications, and there are some. They include dryness of the skin; some chemical imbalances of potassium, magnesium, phosphorus, copper, and proteins; dizziness; fatigue; headache; muscle cramps; rashes; bad breath; diarrhea; or constipation. The most serious one is the possibility of developing irregularities of the heart rate, which may have been responsible for the liquid-protein-diet deaths.

Do these diets work? Well, they often do, particularly on a short-term basis. The weight loss is usually modest, averaging forty-five pounds in one study (but with a gain back of fifteen pounds six months later). There are the usual problems associated with most diet programs. Will the patient remain on the program for the full period of treatment? The appropriate period of time for these drastic diets is twelve to sixteen weeks, followed by three to six weeks of "refeeding" or returning to eating regular food. But even the refeeding period can be dangerous to the health. The second obvious problem is what will happen to the patient's weight after stopping the very-low-calorie diet? The answer, based on most of the reported studies of these programs including Van Itallie and Kral,[11] Bernstein and Van Itallie,[12] and Johnson and Drenick,[13] is dismal. Weight regain can occur as fast as the weight loss. By a year after the diet, a very high percentage of patients regained most or all of their lost weight. Some of these programs are expensive, costing from $2,000 to $3,000.

With such programs as Slimfast® and Dynatrim®, dieters are instructed to drink the powder and skim-milk mixture as a substitute for breakfast and lunch. This provides only 190 to 220 calories per meal. They also offer chocolate bars and puddings containing 100 to 130 calories that the dieter can substitute for the powder and milk mixture. A regular meal, hopefully a relatively low-calorie one, is supposed to be eaten in the evening by the dieter. Thus the actual daily caloric intake is somewhat variable. Apparently, however, most users do not substitute the diet drink for more than half their meals. Many of my patients have felt the drinks were unsatisfactory substitutes for real food, and they were frequently hungry after taking the drinks.

SELF-HELP GROUPS

There are other possibilities for dieting. The so-called self-help groups, or commercial weight-reduction programs have been in existence for forty or fifty years, and have considerable popularity. Of the most popular groups, TOPS, which stands for "Take Off Pounds Sensibly," is probably the oldest, having been started in 1948. Others, including OA (Overeaters Anonymous), WWI (Weight Watchers International), and Diet Workshops began in the 1960s. WWI is the most popular of these, with 43 percent of the market in one study reported in *Consumer Reports*.[14] They are all somewhat different from each other, but there are similarities. OA is essentially based on the principles of Alcoholics Anonymous, and believes that overeating is an addiction similar to alcoholism which, as they say, "can be arrested but not cured." Some of these groups charge a set fee for their program, others are essentially cost-free, except for special foods.

The group setting is a comfortable one for most overweight people, although I have had a few patients say they did not like to spend their time "with a lot of other fat people." New enrollees are given goal weights after their height and weight are measured. Diets are discussed, and in some groups printed diets are handed out. Meetings are held at frequent intervals, usually weekly. Meetings last one to two hours. Members are weighed, and in some groups these are announced aloud for discussion, with praise for weight loss or censure for gain. Nutritional advice may be given, and there may be a lecture by a successful weight-loser, films or tapes, exchange of recipes, singing, and general sharing of experiences.

The groups provide friendly, social, informal settings, peer leaders as role models, and shared experiences, and they generate a faith in the program. They also provide easy entry and withdrawal from the program.

In some of the programs, WWI for example, in addition to weight loss, leveling off and maintenance of lost weight are all covered in the dietary program. Physical activity, support for families, and some aspects of behavior modification may also be part of the group experience. Many enrollees learn what they should be eating, and what not, even if their actual weight loss is minimal.

Some of the commercial programs, such as Jenny Craig®, Nutri/System®, and Physicians Weight Loss Center®, require the purchase and use of company-brand foods. This adds to the cost of the programs, possibly $60 to $70 per week. While exercise is supposed to be encouraged as part of some of these programs, the real emphasis is on decreasing caloric intake.

Success rates seem variable. Even in the same dietary program some groups are more successful than others. Some of this may depend on the effectiveness of the leaders. Dropout rates may be low in the early stages, but they increase as time goes on. Weight loss is relatively small, but most of the enrollees are not massively overweight at the outset. In some groups, average weight losses are about 15 pounds or thereabouts. The very obese and morbidly obese have a greater weight loss in terms of actual pounds, but few reach a satisfactory level. And again, the same problem is present. Weight regain is common, unless active membership is maintained. And even some of the long-term active members regain some or all of their lost weight. In spite of this, I think these groups are good, especially for well-motivated people who only need a relatively small weight reduction.

BEHAVIOR MODIFICATION

Finally, there is behavior modification. These may be the most interesting programs since their goals are to bring about major behavioral changes in the daily way of life of their patients. They make the assumption that obesity is a learning disorder, and that by training an obese patient to behave like a nonobese person weight loss will occur.

Many techniques have been used to accomplish this. Some programs directly attack the eating process. Patients are taught to monitor and regulate their calorie intake. They are instructed to replace their eating utensils back on the table, each time, between bites of food. They are told to eat their meals in only one place, not all over their houses, and television and newspapers are not allowed during meals. In some programs, contracts are made relating to weight losses or gains. For example, with weight loss the enrollee may be paid back part of the original deposit that was put into the program when first enrolling. On the other hand, I have heard of contracts where some of the deposit money goes to the enrollee's most disliked organization or political group if weight is actually gained.

There may be other behavioral aspects covered in these programs. Since, in some patients, overeating may be related to such problems as anxiety, anger, and depression, these issues are addressed by the therapists. An exercise program is often part of the behavior modification treatment. Frequently, husbands and wives of the enrollees are brought into the treatment programs for emotional and social support. In fact, one of the most important aspects of behavior modification is its flexibility in combining its techniques with exercise, weight-loss drugs, and other dietary programs. One program I'm familiar with combines a 520-calorie supplemented diet with a physical activity program, weekly hour-and-a-half educational and behavioral sessions, and weekly physician visits.

EFFECTIVENESS

Do these programs work? The results seem to be variable. In general, the best results occur in patients who are only slightly to moderately obese. There have been some good results in very obese individuals, but more often the weight losses are disappointing. Regain of weight is common, particularly beyond one year after stopping therapy. On the positive side, therapy is safe, with few side effects. And, there are some successes. These programs are relatively new, and there is still much enthusiasm for further development in this field.

So, to sum up, dieting in any form has been disappointing as therapy for those who are overweight and especially for the morbidly obese patient. But diet therapy must be tried by all morbidly obese before any surgery is to be considered. A small number of these patients will be successful, and may not need to be operated on. A friend of mine in Syracuse, a physician, told me he had lost about 100 pounds by dieting and was successfully keeping the weight off. He appeared to be at an ideal weight for his height, and frankly I didn't believe his story. But then later we both attended a hospital dinner party, and while the rest of us were served the usual chicken or roast beef, he was given a huge bowl of lettuce. His wife verified his story. He was living mostly on salads, etc., which probably implied the whole range of foods salads can be made from—vegetables, tuna, chicken, and so on, and his weight remained stable. He told me he had two choices. One, to enjoy himself and eat like everyone else with a gain of 100 pounds, or realize that food would never be one of the enjoyable aspects of his life, and that by living on his salads and the like he could remain healthy and many pounds lighter. He chose the latter. He is truly a rare person!

Consumer Reports magazine, in the June 1993 issue, reported on an extensive survey it conducted on the subject of dieting.[14] Its researchers found that commercial diet programs offered only temporary weight loss for most dieters, the weight loss was usually in the 10 to 20 percent range, and that most regained at least half the weight lost within a year or two. No one program was found to be superior to the others. They reported that a high percentage of dieters were dissatisfied with their program.

In its series on "Fat in America," the *New York Times* in November 1992 noted that commercial diets lack proof of their long-term success. The article suggested that people completing a commercial diet program regain one-third of their lost weight after one year, two-thirds or more after three years, and most, if not all, in three to five years.

Do I have any dieting advice? Not really. I am not a "diet doctor." But I do remember the advice of an old experienced general practitioner from my medical school days. He said, "Tell your patients to diet six days a week, and to eat what they want on the seventh day. This gives them something to look forward to. What they regain on the seventh day will be minimal compared to what they can lose during the six days." This makes good sense to me.

NOTES

1. H. Schwartz, *Never Satisfied* (New York: Free Press, 1986).

2. Ibid.

3. T. B. Van Itallie and J. G. Kral, "The Dilemma of Morbid Obesity," *JAMA* 246 (1981): 999–1003.

4. E. J. Drenick, "Definition and Health Consequences of Morbid Obesity," *Surgical Clinics of North America* 59 (1979): 963–76.

5. T. A. Wadden et al., "The Cambridge Diet," *JAMA* 250 (1983): 2833–34.

6. R. S. Bernstein and T. B. Van Itallie, "An Overview of Therapy for Morbid Obesity," *Surgical Clinics of North America* 59 (1979): 985–94.

7. Van Itallie and Kral, "The Dilemma of Morbid Obesity."

8. Drenick, "Definition and Health Consequences of Morbid Obesity."

9. Bernstein and Van Itallie, "An Overview of Therapy for Morbid Obesity."

10. Wadden et al., "The Cambridge Diet."

11. Van Itallie and Kral, "The Dilemma of Morbid Obesity."

12. Bernstein and Van Itallie, "An Overview of Therapy for Morbid Obesity."

13. D. Johnson and E. J. Drenick, "Therapeutic Fasting in Morbid Obesity," *Archives of Internal Medicine* 137 (1977): 1381–82.

14. *Consumer Reports*, June 1993, pp. 347–57.

10

What About Exercise or Pills?

Who ever hears of fat men heading a riot, or herding together in turbulent mobs?
—Washington Irving, *Knickerbocker's History of New York*

In the last chapter we discussed diets, and more or less concluded that they are not as successful as we would like them to be. Especially for the morbidly obese patients. Here we will discuss treatments that really don't produce long-lasting major weight loss, including exercise, pills, acupuncture, hypnotism, and stomach balloons.

EXERCISE

Now don't get me wrong. I like exercise, and I think it does a lot of good. It just doesn't produce, all by itself, a major loss of weight. Exercise increases the lean-to-fat ratio. In other words, it increases the buildup of muscles. That's very good, but the actual resulting weight loss isn't very great. One study on exercise therapy reported that the average loss of weight was not more than 5 percent of starting weight. While it is true that we burn off more calories during exercise than we do in a resting state, it takes a tremendous amount of activity to lose pounds. Consider the following depressing examples: If you walked all 2,240 steps to the top of the Empire State Building, you would lose half a pound in weight. You would have to lay 14,731 bricks to lose one pound. The calories in one pat of butter are equivalent to climbing all the stairs in the Washington Monument. One donut would equal the calories lost if you conducted an orchestra for two and a half hours. The calories in an ice cream sundae could be burned off by walking five to seven miles.

There are, however, relationships between obesity and the degree of activity. Most studies, including those by Gwinup[1] and Mann,[2] have shown that obese adults are less active than nonobese adults. Of course, the relative inactivity may be a result of the obesity rather than its cause. This appears to be true in children as well, although some studies have shown little difference in physical activity between obese and nonobese children. However, I do remember an old study showing that overweight teenage girls watched much more television than their thinner counterparts. And we probably all remember overweight friends or classmates of ours who seemed "sluggish" or who were not very good ballplayers. You remember, they were the ones who were always picked last when teams were being chosen. On the other hand, I have had several teenage morbidly obese patients who were very athletic in spite of their bulk.

The other uncertainty is whether exercise increases or decreases the appetite. I have seen studies by Gwinup,[3] Pi-Sunyer,[4] Danowski,[5] Oscai et al.,[6] and Krotkiewski et al.[7] giving both answers. Some exercise therapists claim that part of the resulting weight loss after physical exercise is due to a decreased food intake. However, I do know that after I have exercised, like after swimming half a mile, I get extremely hungry. I think this is most people's experience. This may explain an apparent paradox that one of my patients presented. He said he wasn't eating very much, but really wasn't losing very much weight. He was doing a lot of vigorous exercising, lifting weights, and so on. He claimed that his muscle mass was increasing so much that it counteracted any possible weight loss from dieting. I can't accept this. I think he was eating a lot more than he realized, or than he would admit to me.

Although the amount of weight lost after exercising is disappointing, there are obviously many benefits from engaging in a good exercise program. The best programs for burning off calories are those that require movement of the total body mass. These include jogging, walking, swimming, climbing stairs, and cycling. Some of these activities may create major problems for obese individuals who have some physical disabilities, or who may be embarrassed by their appearance when trying to participate with others in a group. The dropout rate in exercise programs is high, possibly in the range of 25 to 75 percent. For some, the routine daily activities, such as walking, using stairs, standing, moving objects, and cleaning, may provide a reasonable amount of exercise.

I strongly urge all of my patients to get into an appropriate exercise program. It helps to rehabilitate them after surgery. They get the feeling that they are returning to a normal life, particularly if their exercise tolerance increases. It's good for them emotionally, and it tightens up muscles and skin. And maybe they do burn off a few extra calories and lose a few extra pounds. Every little bit helps.

WATER CURES

Spas and water cures are another form of physical activity used for all ailments including weight loss. They have always been popular, as far back in history as the ancient Romans and even possibly before. These programs recommended that water be taken internally as well as externally. Various types of baths have been used for trying to lose excess weight. Some of these have included short plunge baths, electric arc light baths, cold rain douches, sweating packs, cold dripping sheets, and steam baths. Spas and the baths are still popular today and they continue to "cure" all ailments. How effective they are for losing weight remains a very good question.

WEIGHT-REDUCING DRUGS

Now let's move to weight-reducing drugs or pills. Patent medicines for weight loss have been available for years in many forms and varieties. They have included cathartics, emetics, diuretics (water pills), laxatives, digitalis (as a stimulant), camphor (supposedly an appetite suppressant), thyroid, arsenic, strychnine, caffeine, pokeberry (an emetic and purgative), and many others. There were Densmore's Corpulency Cure (sassafras tea), Slenderine, Richard Hudnut's Obesity Pills, Chichester's Corpus Lean, and Dr. Gordon's Elegant Pills.

Somebody is making a lot of money from these pills, and most just don't work very well. There were several studies from the University of Michigan and Michigan State University[8] a few years ago that pointed out the extensive use of these medications. One study showed that 40 percent of high school girls have used weight-reduction pills, and another study showed that 30 percent of college-age women had used them. A quarter of these women reported side effects from the pills. Also, about half of the women were taking doses twice or three times the dose recommended by the manufacturer. Now, with all this extensive use you would expect some positive results, wouldn't you? But 86 percent of the women who used the pills said they were not effective over the long term, or had little or no effect on suppressing appetite, or were totally ineffective.

The "modern era" probably started with the use of thyroid extract in the 1890s. These preparations became available over the counter without prescription. Such preparations as Safe Fat Reducer, Marmola, Newman's Obesity Cure, Corpulin, Elimiton, Phy-thy-rin, San-Gri-Na, and Trilene all contained thyroid or iodine components. All of these tried to raise the body's metabolic rate and burn off calories. They do produce some loss of weight. But doses within the range of *ordinary* daily requirements of thyroid hormone are ineffective for weight loss.

Relatively high doses are needed and that's when the side effects begin. These include all the symptoms of an overactive thyroid, including chest pain, increased heart rate, palpitations, sweating, heat intolerance, and general nervousness—all of which are very unpleasant and actually quite dangerous. It's amazing that thyroid medicines are still being given to patients to produce weight loss, in spite of their ineffectiveness and the dangers. The so-called sluggish thyroids of obese patients should be proved or disproved by thyroid function tests before administering medication. If the thyroid proves to be underactive, thyroid hormone replacement therapy should be prescribed. Otherwise not.

Since an increase in metabolic rate does burn off body fat, much interest has been generated in finding other drugs that might work this way. Dinitrophenol is one of these drugs. It has been around since the 1880s, but was first used for weight loss around 1933. In such preparations as Corpu-lean and Formula 37, it increases the metabolic rate and burns off fat, with a weight loss of as much as 2 to 3 pounds per week. But this is an extremely toxic and dangerous drug. With its increase in body-heat production, users feel warm, perspire, develop rashes, lose taste, develop cataracts, and because of the high body temperatures some go into comas and die. Needless to say, this drug was stopped in 1938 and is no longer available.

Just as Dinitrophenol was discontinued, the first of the amphetamines, Dexedrine, became available. Because of the undesirable side effects, a variety of related compounds has been synthesized. Currently available are Desoxyn, Biphetamine, and Didrex. Although they appear to be appetite suppressants, the exact mechanism of action is not known. The greatest weight loss occurs during the first few weeks, and it isn't all that much. The drugs become less and less effective, and there is the tendency to increase the dosage, in spite of the warnings not to do so. As everyone knows, there is a high potential for abuse of amphetamines and drug dependency can occur. Furthermore, these are very dangerous drugs from a medical point of view. Patients with heart disease, high blood pressure, overactive thyroids, glaucoma, or history of drug abuse are not supposed to use amphetamines. Side effects include insomnia, agitation, dizziness, tremor, headache, impotence, hallucinations, elevation of blood pressure, palpitations, rapid heart rate, and others. Permission to use these drugs for weight loss has been cut back by many states. For a while, New York State permitted use for only a one-month period. But since about 1981 it has been illegal for physicians in New York to prescribe amphetamines for weight loss.

There is a newer group of drugs that are considered nonamphetamines but have actions similar to the amphetamines group. These include Adipex, Bontril, Fastin, Ionamin, Plegine, Prelu-2, Sanorex, and Tenuate. While the incidence of side effects may be somewhat lower, the potential dangers still exist. Users develop tolerance to the drugs and they become even less effective fairly quickly. Manufacturers recommend only short-term use at most. Weight loss is not impressive.

PHEN/FEN

Pondimin (fenfluramine) was FDA-approved many years ago. In 1995, dexfenfluramine was approved by the FDA, the first antiobesity drug in about twenty-three years. It was marketed under the name Redux. These drugs alter brain levels of a drug called *serotonin* to make people feel full even when they have eaten less. Their use was aimed at the very obese, those 30 percent over their ideal weight or those 20 percent over ideal weight if they also had obesity-related medical complications. From the very beginning of their use, there were questions about their safety. Weight loss was relatively modest and the drugs were to be used by patients in conjunction with dieting. Short-term use had relatively poor results, but there were few studies on the safety of long-term use.

However, all this did not stop the very extensive use of these drugs, which were considered to be wonder drugs. The combination of fenflu-ramine and phentermine resin, the so-called phen/fen drugs, and Redux had tremendous sales, even among those only slightly overweight. For example, in 1996, about 18 million prescriptions were written for phen/fen. Some of the commercial diet centers, such as NutriSystem® and Jenny Craig® used the drugs in some patients along with dieting. But the complications were being reported: primary pulmonary hypertension, a potentially lethal condition, was found to be ten times greater in users of these drugs, and supposedly more than twenty times greater with use of these drugs for more than three months. Heart valve damage was reported in as many as 30 percent of those taking the drugs. As a result, the FDA requested in September of 1997 that these drugs be withdrawn from the market, and the pharmaceutical companies stopped making Redux and fenfluramine available. Some doctors have substituted Prozac for fenfluramine, giving patients the phen/Pro combination. One of the side effects of Prozac is loss of appetite, although Eli Lilly, the company that makes Prozac, has not endorsed the use of this drug for weight loss.

Currently available for weight loss is Meridia (sibutramine). This drug supposedly increases the feeling of fullness and speeds up the rate the body burns up calories. Weight loss appears to be modest though the drug is used with dieting and exercise. Much is still not known about this drug, especially in its long-term use. However, it is known to increase blood pressure in some patients and regular monitoring of blood pressure may be necessary.

OVER-THE-COUNTER DRUGS

The next group of drugs are probably the most popular of all. These are the over-the-counter drugs, those that can be bought without a prescrip-tion. I found the following in my local drugstore: Acutrim®, Permathene-12®, Appedrine®, Prolamine®, and Dexatrim®. The active ingredient in all of these is phenylpropanolamine, which is also a derivative of amphet-amine. But side effects seem to be less common and less serious. We're advised not to use these drugs if we have high blood pressure, depression, heart disease, diabetes, or thyroid disease. As with all of the above, weight loss with this group of medications is fairly low grade.

OTHERS

The story only gets worse. Diuretics, or water pills, such as Lasix do produce short-lived weight loss. This is obviously related to water loss. Weight is rapidly regained as body water is replaced. Furthermore, diuretics are potentially dangerous if used in conjunction with fasting.

Chorionic Gonadotropin was first used for weight loss in 1954. It's supposed to just melt away fat and help the user tolerate low-calorie diets better. The most recent carefully conducted studies by Shetty and Kalkhoff[9] and Young and associates[10] clearly show that this drug is not at all effective. Another hormone, dehydroepiandrosterone or DHEA, supposedly produced weight loss, prolonged life, and enhanced sexual performance. None of these claims were ever proven. The Food and Drug Administration stopped the sale of this drug in the 1980s.

The so-called bulking agents, such as methycellulose and guar gum, are supposed to decrease food intake by stretching the stomach wall. They do not appear to be very effective. One problem is that they swell up only very slowly, usually after leaving the stomach and reaching the intestines.

There are numerous drugs that have been tried and discarded, or tried and should be discarded. Digitalis, the heart medicine, was used to control the rapid pulse rate that occurred when thyroid hormone was given for weight loss. While overdoses of digitalis do suppress the appetite, there is no safe or rational reason to use it for this purpose.

So at the present time, diet pills do not offer the obese individual an easy, safe, and effective way of getting rid of the excess weight. This could change eventually. The rules are well defined. The ideal drug must significantly reduce body weight, have long-term effects without tolerance developing, not result in a weight regain when discontinued, and have no undesirable side effects.

ACUPUNCTURE

With the drug approach proving ineffective, those desperate for weight loss turn to more unusual methods. One such avenue is acupuncture. This is an Asiatic technique of placing needles at specific points in the skin to produce the desired effect. This has been used for the control of pain in China for a long time, but the use of acupuncture for weight loss is fairly new. The ear is used, because, as I understand it, it is like a human body in a partially curled up position. Needles or stainless steel staples are placed in the part of the ear representing the stomach or mouth. The use of staples apparently eliminates the need for putting needles in the ear each time the patient feels hungry; the staples are kept in the ear for a long time. I have been told by patients who have had this done that they were supposed to press or squeeze the staple when they feel hungry, and that was supposed to relieve the hunger. I have seen this technique referred to as *auriculotherapy*. Does it work? I haven't seen too much written about it in scientific journals, but one study by Mok and colleagues[11] that seemed to be done in a careful manner did not show any weight loss from the treatment. I have had several patients who had had acupuncture treatments for weight loss, and all had failed. The staples I have seen used were relatively large, and looked like wood staples. I have wondered whether infections occur as a result of this nonsterile placement in the ear, but apparently they are uncommon. One patient did say that when she squeezed the staple as directed her ear hurt. But it did not hurt enough to stop eating. When we performed her gastric bypass we also removed the staple.

HYPNOTISM

I really don't know much about hypnotism. It has been used to treat obesity and overeating, but I have not been able to find any medical studies on its effectiveness. Through the years I have had a number of patients who have tried hypnosis, but none has had much success. One patient told me that its effects lasted for ten minutes. When I asked her what she meant by that, she replied, "I didn't feel like eating for ten minutes after I left the hypnosis session. Then I passed a pizza parlor . . ."

GASTRIC BALLOON

The most recent approach for treating obesity started in about 1985. This was the *gastric balloon*. Some years before this, I remember a sort of joke that was going around in medical circles about a treatment for obesity. "You put a balloon in the patient's stomach. Whenever the patient feels hungry, you inflate the balloon with air, the hunger goes away, and the patient loses weight." Sure enough, someone took this seriously and the gastric balloon was invented. A deflated plastic balloon shaped like a cylinder is passed into the stomach by way of a tube inserted through the mouth. The balloon is then inflated with air and detached from the tube. The balloon is about the size and shape of a small frozen orange juice can. It apparently takes up about 20 to 30 percent of the space in the stomach. The balloon is left in the stomach for four months and then removed, after deflation, by a tube inserted into the stomach through the mouth.

The patients treated with balloon therapy appeared to eat less and lost weight. Nobody is certain why the weight loss occurs since the stomach is not fully occupied or distended by the balloon. There was a lot of excitement about this technique and a lot of publicity.

A number of questions were raised. What happens to the patients after removing the balloon? Do they regain any lost weight? The balloon doctors tell us that the balloons can be reinserted for a second four-month period, and even for a third period. All well and good, but sooner or later the balloon treatment would have to be stopped. What then? We are told that the patients by that time have learned good eating habits, and would never again overeat and regain their weight. I remained skeptical about these claims and patiently waited for some long-term follow-up studies. Based on my experience with gastric-bypass patients, I couldn't believe that removing the balloon would be followed by stable weight. Sometimes the staples would come apart in gastric-bypass patients and there would no longer be a physical barrier limiting the amount of food that could be eaten. I found out that the patients "learned" nothing, and started eating again as much as before the surgery, even if this occurred several years after the operation. I didn't believe that the "balloon" patients would "learn" anything either.

There were also questions relating to the actual effectiveness of balloons in terms of weight loss. In one good investigation by Mathus-Vliegen et al.,[12] a so-called randomized, prospective, double-blind, crossover study (which is the most scientific, nonbiased type of study), patients were not told whether a balloon was actually put in or not. Patients having the sham procedure (no balloon) lost as much weight as the balloon patients since they were all put on a very-low-calorie diet. In a study by Yang and associates[13] using experimental animals (pigs), none of the animals lost weight with the balloons.

But since this seemed like such a good way to lose weight, the technique became very popular. Supposedly 17,000 balloons were put in patients in the first year after the balloons were given approval by the

Food and Drug Administration. Unfortunately, as more balloons were used, the complications began to appear. And these complications were very serious. The balloons sometimes irritated the lining of the stomach, causing abrasions and actual ulcers of the stomach, occasionally with bleeding. Perforation of the stomach could also occur, or perforation of the esophagus as the balloon was being removed. Or, if the balloon became deflated, it could obstruct the lower end of the stomach or the intestine as it began to pass through the digestive tract. All of these were very serious problems, life threatening, and frequently required major operations. The suggested time for keeping the balloon in the stomach was reduced from four months to three months, but the problems continued.

The gastric balloon quickly lost favor and has been withdrawn from production. It belongs now only to the history books.

It's obvious that exercise, diet pills, or gimmicks are not the answer to morbid obesity. I find the situation with diet pills particularly depressing. So many things have been tried and there still is no "magic bullet." Perhaps someday. It is also depressing to see how long the history of morbid obesity is. We sometimes think of it as a twentieth-century phenomenon, but as you have seen, it has a history of its own.

NOTES

1. G. Gwinup, "Effects of Diet and Exercise," in G. A. Bray and G. E. Bethune, *Treatment and Management of Obesity* (Hagerstown, Md.: Harper & Row, 1974), pp. 93–102.

2. G. V. Mann, "The Influence of Obesity in Health, Part 1," *New England Journal of Medicine* 291 (1974): 178–85.

3. Gwinup, "Effects of Diet and Exercise."

4. F. X. Pi-Sunyer, "Exercise Effects on Caloric Intake," in R. J . Wurtman and J. J. Wurtman, *Human Obesity* (New York: New York Academy of Sciences, 1987), 94–103.

5. T. S. Danowski, "The Management of Obesity," *Hospital Practice* (1976): 39–44.

6. L. B. Oscai et al., "Exercise or Food Restriction: Effect on Adipose Tissue Cellularity," *American Journal of Physiology* 227 (1974): 901–904.

7. M. Krotkiewski et al., "Effects of Long-Term Physical Training on Body Fat, Metabolism and Blood Pressure in Obesity," *Metabolism* 28 (1979): 650–58.

8. "Studies Show Popularity of Diet Pills," in *American Medical News* (1984), quoting from the University of Michigan and Michigan State University studies.

9. K. R. Shetty and R. K. Kalkhoff, "Human Chorionic Gonadotropin (HCG) Treatment of Obesity," *Archives of Internal Medicine* 137 (1977): 151–55.

10. R. L. Young, R. J. Fuchs, and M. J. Woltjen, "Chorionic Gonadotropin in Weight Control," *JAMA* 236 (1976): 2495–97.

11. M. S. Mok et al., "Treatment of Obesity by Acupuncture," *American Journal of Clinical Nutrition* 29 (1976): 832–35.

12. E. M. H. Mathus-Vliegen, G. N. J. Tytgat, and E. A. M. L. Veldhuyzen-Offermans, "Intragastric Balloon in the Treatment of Super-Morbid Obesity," *Gastroenterology* 99 (1990): 362–69.

13. Y. Yang et al., "Use of Intragastric Balloons for Weight Reduction," *American Journal of Surgery* 153 (1987): 265–69.

11

Intestinal Bypass: My Syracuse Experience

It is the part of a wise man to feed himself with moderate pleasant food and drink.

—Spinoza, *Ethics*

I moved to Syracuse in the summer of 1974. My job as professor of surgery at the Upstate Medical Center, part of the State University of New York, included the clinical practice of surgery, teaching medical students and surgical residents, and continuing my research on blood circulation in animal cancers. The combination of clinical practice, teaching, and research are sometimes considered the "three-legged stool" characteristic of so-called academic surgery. In addition, there was the now-inevitable administrative work that included committee participation, paperwork of all sorts, and so on. I spent part of my time at the university hospital, in the medical center, and part at the Syracuse Veterans Hospital, which was only a block or so away.

As a general surgeon, I operated at both hospitals doing surgery on the stomach, small and large intestine, liver, gallbladder, pancreas, spleen, breast, and other organs considered to be the territory of the general surgeon. Of course I intended to continue my interest in morbid obesity. But getting started with this took a little time. Some intestinal bypasses for the extremely overweight had been done there before I moved to Syracuse, and apparently many had not gone well. Some doctors at the hospital had serious doubts about operating on morbidly obese people, and I ran into some resistance. On the other hand, I expressed a reasonable amount of confidence based on my favorable, although somewhat limited, experience. Happily, we met each other half way.

It was agreed that these operations were to be considered a sort of research project, and that there would be frequent meetings, reviews, and evaluations by all those interested. I had no objection to this, although it was really not "research" in any sense of the word. After all, many thousands of these operations had already been done all over the world, and done safely. But my colleagues at the medical center wanted to make absolutely sure it could be done safely at our hospitals. A committee was set up to develop a protocol, which would include the rules and regulations under which I would select patients for these operations and the preoperative tests that would have to be done. At a university, there's always a committee! And you know how they function. Dr. Wangensteen, my chief of surgery at the University of Minnesota, would often say, "If Moses had had a committee, he would still be waiting for the Red Sea to part."

But things moved along, and the rules were reasonable. Suggestions for the preoperative testing were fairly extensive. After all, my committee included endocrinologists, gastroenterologists, internists, a psychiatrist, a pathologist, surgeons, and a few others. The tests agreed upon were a complete blood count, urinalysis, chest X-ray, liver function blood tests, serum electrolyte levels (sodium, potassium, chloride, and carbonate), serum calcium, phosphate and magnesium levels, serum iron levels, thyroid and adrenal function tests, serum lipid profiles (cholesterol and triglycerides), a 3-to-4-hour glucose tolerance test for diabetes, an electrocardiogram, pulmonary function tests, arterial blood gases, a gallbladder X-ray, sometimes a kidney X-ray, and a whole variety of intestinal absorption tests and serum vitamin levels. That's quite a list. I actually did not understand why we needed some of these tests, but the committee was happy. Fortunately, after a year of experience with good results, the committee was satisfied that the operations would be done safely on the appropriate patients. I then eliminated the tests that I thought were unnecessary and streamlined things a bit.

This all happened in the mid-1970s during the "good old days." Patients living near Syracuse were admitted to the hospital three to five days before surgery to finish up the tests. Those living farther away were actually admitted five days before surgery to do the testing. Today, we would never be allowed to admit patients for testing. Everything has to be done as an outpatient. While this makes sense fiscally, it does put a major strain on very heavy, disabled, arthritic patients who have terrible difficulties getting from one place to another.

For readers who may have noticed that psychological testing and evaluation were not on our routine preoperative list, these tests did not seem to be helpful unless there were specific psychological indications for them, in the experience of most surgeons doing intestinal bypasses. Our group agreed. We were fortunate to have Dr. Ellen Cook working with us. She had been an internist, was now a psychiatrist, and had much experience working with both obese and anorexic patients. She agreed that evaluation of these morbidly obese patients was difficult, and that predicting which ones might develop emotional problems after surgery was very inaccurate, even for her. She was a tremendous help to me in those few instances when psychiatric help was really needed.

All this setting up took time. My first intestinal bypass in Syracuse was in February 1975. Referral of patients to me was slow at first. My initial source of patients was from our surgical clinics and from other surgeons. Some referrals were from our orthopedic surgeons (patients with back and hip problems), neurosurgeons, gynecologists, and psychiatrists. Our patients who had good results started to refer their friends who were morbidly obese, and also family members. Then, surgeons in surrounding communities who heard that we were doing these operations at the medical center began to send us their patients. Soon I was very busy. Interestingly enough, it took a very long time before my internal-medicine colleagues recognized the value of the operations and referred their patients. My surgical friends reassured me by quoting the Bible, "A prophet is not without honor, save in his own country, and in his own house."

All new patients met with me for an hour or so to discuss all aspects of the operation I was proposing. We talked about the preoperative tests, the operation and how it was done, the time spent in the hospital, possible postoperative complications, expected weight loss, and other benefits. Questions were asked and answered. These questions covered various concerns, such as the success rate of the operation, would their insurance cover the cost of the operation, when would weight loss start, and so forth. I then asked my patients some questions about the onset of their obesity, family history of obesity, existing medical or emotional problems, previous operations, medications, allergies, attempts to diet, etc.

When I became fairly busy after a few years, I began to have discussions with groups of patients, rather than with just one patient at a time. This made it easier for me, and the patients liked it better, too. They discovered that they were not alone in this world, and that others had similar problems with their weight. Also, if one patient was reluctant to ask certain questions, there was always another one present who was not so reluctant. The sessions were often noisy, sometimes raucous, and a good camaraderie frequently developed.

The five or six morbidly obese patients attending these sessions often brought relatives and friends with them, and some of these people were also very heavy. Some of my surgical associates said that the hospital seemed to lean to one side on the days when I had these sessions. I didn't think that was too funny, but sometimes amusing things did occur. One day I was a little late arriving at the session with the patients. As I walked in the door they all started to laugh. They said, "None of us has ever seen you before. We only spoke to you over the phone. We decided that if you were as fat as we are, we were all going to leave." I realized then that keeping thin was a career necessity for me.

Most of the patients I saw were from around the Syracuse area. But eventually my patients were from as far north as Lake Ontario, as far south as the Pennsylvania border area, westward almost to Rochester, and eastward almost to Albany. In other words, the central part of New York State. There were a few towns or small cities in this area that seemed to send me relatively large numbers of patients. I have heard similar comments from surgeons in other parts of the country. There just seem to be some obesity-prone cities and towns. For me, it was Oswego and Mexico, New York. Maybe it had something to do with the cold weather up there.

Most of my patients were admitted to one particular surgical floor at the Upstate Medical Center. At first, the nurses had a lot of doubts about this. The usual comment was "Why don't they just go on a diet and lose the weight? Why do they have to have to come in the hospital and have an operation?" I did a lot of talking to the nurses for the first few years which helped the situation somewhat. But what really made the difference was the patients themselves. The nurses began to realize how unhappy and unhealthy the patients were, and how they changed when weight loss occurred. Many of the patients came back to visit the nurses six months or a year after the operation. Some of the patients had changed so much with the loss of weight that they were unrecognizable by the nurses. The patients had to bring before-and-after pictures so that the nurses could remember them. The whole thing got to be pretty funny at times. You'd hear comments like "No, that can't possibly be you!" and "Oh, now I remember you, but I don't believe it!" and so on. What finally developed was a good close relationship between the nurses, patients, and me.

There were a few nurses and also one housekeeper in the hospital who were very negative at first. Apparently someone on the floor would tell some of the patients the night before the operation that they should leave before it was too late because they probably were going to die. As you can imagine, the patients weren't too happy about this, and they complained to me and to the head nurses. I had trouble believing that anyone in the hospital would actually say such things to my patients but apparently it happened. It just shows how emotional this whole subject of morbid obesity can become sometimes. I eventually talked to the nurses and other workers and the problem seemed to resolve itself.

The operation I performed was the same one that I had done in Kansas City: connecting the first 12 inches of jejunum to the last 8 inches of ileum, in an end-to-end fashion, bypassing about 90 percent of the total length of the small intestine. There was still a lot of discussion going on about how much jejunum and ileum to use, and how to connect them. I didn't make any changes in the operation, since it seemed to be working satisfactorily.

The first operations I performed in Syracuse were somewhat exciting. Most of the nurses and doctors had never seen such heavy patients, nor had they seen any such operations. But after a while, it became "routine." I still remember those first patients even though it's been more than twenty years. They will always be special since they were really a beginning for me. Some of them were especially memorable. There was one lovely woman, Mary, who had a very kind, attentive husband. She had been referred to me because of her very severe back pain, apparently related to her obesity. She had a pretty good result from the operation, and about a year later was able to dance and play golf. I frequently told later patients about this, but I was always careful to say that I didn't guarantee anything about dancing and golfing.

Another one of those early patients was an exceptionally heavy young woman, Susan, weighing about 480 pounds. She had a hernia around her navel (an umbilical hernia) and some of her internal organs were stuck in the hernia. She would sometimes fall and land on this area of the hernia. We were afraid that part of her small intestine might be stuck in the hernia, and that this would burst when she fell on it. Also, she occasionally became stuck in her bathtub (like William Howard Taft) and the volunteer fire department in her town would have to come and pull her out. I operated on her and the surgery went well. The defect around the navel causing the hernia was very small, but there was a grapefruit-sized wad of omentum (the intra-abdominal fat pad) that was caught in the hernia. It was impressive. But when I removed this omentum, I found it weighed only 4 pounds. I then realized that fat itself is not so heavy, and that it is the muscles, bones, etc., that account for the weight. Remember, fat floats on water; think of droplets of oil floating on the surface of water.

I should mention that in these operations we didn't just do the bypassing of the intestines. We almost always performed a liver biopsy, that is, removal of a very small piece of liver, which was then processed and looked at under a microscope by the pathologists. Most of the patients had some abnormality of the liver, although usually not serious. It was usually infiltration of fat into the liver, with some slight degree of inflammation. Since we worried about the changes in the liver that occurred later after the operation, sometimes we did a percutaneous liver biopsy six or twelve months later. This involved sticking a special needle through the skin and abdominal wall, with the use of local anesthesia, down to the liver itself. A small core of liver tissue was removed and given to the pathologists. In the case of the woman described above, her liver tissue at six months after surgery was so infiltrated with fat that it actually floated on the formaldehyde solution in which it was placed. She fortunately had enough normal functioning liver tissue present, and she had no problems from this. Twelve months after the surgery, her liver was normal.

During these operations we also removed the patient's appendix since appendicitis is relatively common in this age group. Any abnormalities that we found during an exploration of the abdomen were also taken care of. The most common of these abnormalities were gallstones and hernias of the navel.

12

Benefits of Intestinal Bypass

Open thine eyes, and thou shalt be satisfied with bread.
—Proverbs (Bible)

From 1975 to 1982, I performed intestinal bypass operations on about 150 morbidly obese patients. They ranged in age from seventeen to fifty-three years, with an average age of thirty-six years. Women outnumbered men about three to one. The patients all weighed more than 100 pounds over their ideal weights, with a range of 213 to 579 pounds. The average patient weighed 321 pounds. Almost all of them had medical or physical complaints that were related to their extreme obesity. About a third had high blood pressure. Diabetes was also common. Almost a third of the patients had at least a slightly abnormal blood sugar level. Fifteen of these patients were actually diabetics requiring daily insulin injections or pills. Nearly half of the morbidly obese patients complained of back pain or arthritis, mainly involving their hips, knees, and ankles. Another common problem was hyperlipemia, with almost one-third having increased levels of serum cholesterol or triglycerides. Finally, gallbladder disease was also very common. About 40 percent had this problem, but two-thirds of them already had had their gallbladder removed before coming to see me. I removed the gallbladders of eighteen patients when I performed their intestinal bypasses.

Although some of the operations were fairly difficult, particularly on some of the heaviest patients, virtually all went through the operation without serious problems. For the first few days after the operation they were not allowed to eat or drink, and they received only intravenous fluids. When some of the patients asked me how soon they would start to lose weight, I would answer "Immediately!" They couldn't eat at first because the intestinal suture lines had to heal, and it took a few days for the intestine to regain its normal propulsive activity. Also, they all had a nasogastric tube, a long tube extending from outside the nose down into the stomach, which sucked out any air or fluid in the stomach. After about three days, we removed this tube. Then they were started on liquids by mouth, and finally regular food. Most patients were able to leave the hospital in about a week.

The postoperative period was not easy for most patients. Just about all of the patients had diarrhea. The degree of the diarrhea, how many bowel movements per day, was the only issue. But before we go into that, let's talk about the positive side of the operation. All patients lost weight. Sometimes it was very good. Sometimes it was fantastic!

WHY DID THEY LOSE WEIGHT?

The question often came up, why did they lose all that weight? The obvious answer was that with only 10 percent of their small intestine actually functioning they were absorbing only a fraction of the calories that they were eating. And there was good evidence that they were not absorbing everything they swallowed. Malabsorption of protein, for example, seemed to be the cause of a very serious problem, liver dysfunction, in a small number of patients. We'll discuss this more later. The bowel movements often had unabsorbed fat in them. Calcium, potassium, and magnesium were sometimes poorly absorbed, and this produced other problems. Also, the fat soluble vitamins, A, D, and E, were not absorbed well. Finally, some medicines were imperfectly absorbed which produced some interesting consequences. For example, birth-control pills were not always completely absorbed. One surgeon told me of a patient who unexpectedly found herself pregnant, and not too happy about it. After hearing about that, I instructed my female patients to consider other means of birth control, at least for a year or so. Of more immediate peril, some heart and epilepsy medications were poorly absorbed, and substitutions had to be made.

In spite of this evidence, some researchers insisted that the patients lost weight simply because they ate less after the surgery. And why did they eat less? These researchers replied that the patients came to realize that if they ate less the terrible diarrhea would decrease. I strongly doubt this. Weight loss appeared to be unrelated to the degree of diarrhea, and none of my patients said that they ate less in order to control the diarrhea, even when asked about it. But they did eat less. I did not instruct them to decrease their caloric intake, but they did so spontaneously.

In a study we conducted, we found that three months after surgery they were eating about 3,000 calories a day, which was about half of their preoperative 6,000-to-7,000-calorie intake. But the other factor, malabsorption of calories, was also apparent. Compare their 3000-calorie intake, three months after surgery, to that of the gastric-bypass patients. The gastric-bypass patients three months after their operations were only eating 740 calories per day. Now both groups of patients were losing a similar amount of weight. (Actually this intestinal-bypass group was losing a little more weight.) The only way that the intestinal-bypass group could have such a weight loss was that some of the calories were not being absorbed. Also, when intestinal bypasses were performed on experimental animals such as rats, weight loss did occur. Now rats would not be expected to modify their eating habits just to control their diarrhea. But they did eat less. So what's the answer? I think the weight loss after intestinal bypass was due to two factors. First, the patients absorbed calories poorly because of their shortened small intestine. Second, they ate less because of a decrease in appetite, although they still packed away a lot of calories. We don't totally understand the mechanisms of appetite and its control. Apparently there is an intestinal phase of appetite that can be modified by shortening the length of the intestine.

How Much Weight Loss?

How much weight did these patients actually lose? Before I go into this, I should explain how I determine such weight loss. Some surgeons calculate the percent loss of *excess* weight. In other words, they say that the patients are so many pounds heavier than their ideal weight, and when they lose weight, the surgeons divide the pounds lost by the number of pounds originally above the established ideal weight. I've never liked this. There is really no one single number that can be called one's ideal weight. Instead, ideal weight is generally expressed as a range of pounds. So which number should be used in the calculation? It seems very arbitrary to me. I've preferred to stick to the actual weights themselves. The patient starts with a certain weight and loses some pounds. The pounds lost divided by the original weight equals the *percent weight lost.* Simple and totally honest.

The average weight loss of my patients has been 38 percent of the starting weight. But there is a very wide range of percent weight loss, going way up to 65 percent of the starting weight! I consider a weight loss of 25 percent or more as a success. About 92 percent of my patients are successful by this standard. And 97 percent lose at least 20 percent of their starting weight. The older patients did as well as the younger ones, and the men lost slightly more, but this is probably not statistically significant. In my early surgeries, there was one interesting finding. The percent of weight loss appeared to be directly related to the actual preoperative weight. The weight loss of patients weighing less than 250 pounds averaged 30 percent. My "superobese" patients, weighing more than 400 pounds before surgery, lost an average of 50 percent. Weight loss was rapid during the first few months after surgery, then it slowed down, and finally stopped somewhere between twelve to eighteen months. The period of weight loss for the "superobese" group often went on for twenty-four months and beyond.

PATIENTS' STORIES

Now those are the numbers. But what does all of this actually mean to the patient? Let me tell some of their stories.

One very nice patient of mine, Amy, was in her mid-thirties and weighed about 330 pounds. She had high blood pressure; arthritis in her back, knees, and ankles; and possible diabetes. She had a good family and a very supportive husband. After her intestinal bypass she had some of the complications associated with it (diarrhea and low potassium, calcium, and magnesium), but gradually improved. Her weight continued to go down, and finally leveled off about eighteen months after surgery. Her lowest weight was recorded at 175 pounds, which was a 48 percent weight loss. Since she was 5 feet 8 inches tall, her new weight was quite satisfactory. Around Christmas or New Year's after she had lost most of the weight, her husband took her "out on the town" for dinner and dancing. Several days later, she received two confidential phone calls from friends who hadn't seen her since the operation. Both friends told her that they had seen her husband out with another woman. . . . It was her! Or the *new* her. That's what often happens. It becomes very hard to recognize the patient after such a major weight loss.

Another one of my favorite patients was a very nice thirty-year-old high school teacher, Sam. He weighed over 400 pounds. He also had high blood pressure and some arthritis. The intestinal bypass went very well, and he had almost no postoperative problems. When I saw him last about four years after surgery, his weight was 229 pounds, a 49 percent loss. About seventeen years after his operation, I heard from his wife. He had been married for about twelve years and had several children. The operation was a success.

Talking about successes, one of my young female patients, Sarah, who weighed over 480 pounds dropped her weight down after surgery to a low point of 177 pounds, a 63 percent weight loss. She looked great at her new weight. She then got married, had a few children, and started raising her family. Unfortunately, she later divorced. Clearly not all problems are solved by weight loss.

Many of the young women who had good weight losses really looked good, a few even looked terrific. Some told me that their husbands became much more attentive than they had been in years. One woman, Beth, said that when she and her husband now go together to a shopping mall, her husband puts his arm around her waist. When I asked her how she and her husband walked before her operation, she replied, "He was always six feet in front of me." Many husbands became very protective and became jealous if another man looked at their wife. One husband who was a long-distance truck driver started to take his wife on the trips with him.

Those were the good husbands. Not all were good. One of my female patients, Jean, was forty years old and weighed about 325 pounds before surgery. After the intestinal-bypass surgery, she had many complications and eventually was reoperated on. I converted her operation to a gastric bypass, but still she had problems. Finally she improved and her weight dropped to 135 pounds. At that point, her husband left her for a younger woman—a twenty-year-old, who weighed 300 pounds! Who could have imagined it!

MARRIAGE AND DIVORCE

Actually, divorces were fairly common. But usually it was the now slimmed-down woman who instituted the proceedings. It was commonly a "Jack Spratt and wife" situation. These very heavy women sometimes had small, often runty men. Some men cheated on their wives, abused them, and took all their money. Some husbands blurted out that their wives were lucky to get any man, even them. Well, these women had surgery, lost weight, looked at themselves in the mirror, looked at their husbands, and then they said to themselves, "I can do better than this" and got a divorce. That's what an improved self-image can do. Rand, Kuldau, and Robbins,[1] a group of psychiatrists, conducted a study on this and found that some of these woman had, among other things, increased sexuality. Apparently some husbands couldn't keep up with their wives in this regard, and this also led to marital breakups.

One last story about marriage. One of my female patients, Patricia, told me that she and her husband joked about how good she was going to look after her operation, and that he wanted her to sign a paper guaranteeing that she would not leave him when she became thin and beautiful. They laughed about this. Then she had her operation, lost a lot of weight, and—you guessed it—she divorced him.

MORE PATIENTS' STORIES

My male patients were certainly no Jack Spratts. They were big and heavy, averaging almost 400 pounds. One winter, I had quite a spate of very heavy male patients—five of them—all weighing from about 400 to 500 pounds. And all were married to small, thin, and attractive women. Most of them had children, and I always wondered how these small women with very large husbands managed to get pregnant. Or what position they used. Think about it.

Most of my male patients were very pleasant individuals. Three were high school teachers, one was the manager of traveling carnival shows, and several were businessmen. The heaviest was Edward, a twenty-two-year-old weighing 579 pounds. Medically, he was in amazingly good health, except for some pains in his knees. His intestinal bypass went well, and he progressed exceptionally well afterward. According to my records, he weighed about 240 pounds two years after his operation—a 58 percent weight loss! His older brother, George, who I also operated on, weighed 514 pounds. His results were also quite good, and his weight dropped down to the low 200s. One other young man I operated on, William, always came to my office with his mother. Although I'm sure she meant well, she was always very critical of her 470-pound son, saying things about him—in his presence—that I thought were awful. After he started to lose a lot of weight, he seemed to break free of her, came to see me alone, and did some traveling on his own. I felt very good about this, and hoped his mother realized how much healthier it was for him to be on his own. The last time I saw him, about two years after his operation, he weighed 195 pounds, a 58 percent weight loss.

One of the heaviest women I operated on, Sylvia, weighed 492 pounds, but was only 5 feet $1\frac{1}{2}$ inches tall. She suffered from a massive thickening of the skin of her lower legs, and the skin was hanging in rolls around her legs. On one leg there was a big grapefruit-sized mass of thickened skin, which prevented her from putting her two legs together. She walked with a wobbly, clumsy gait. Her weight loss was the most spectacular in terms of percentages. After two years she had lost 329 pounds, achieving a weight of 163 pounds. This was a 67 percent loss. With such weight reduction the redundant skin on her legs really hung down. She underwent plastic surgery for this problem, and while it didn't look beautiful, it was very functional. And for the first time in years she could walk with her legs close together in a normal fashion. Just imagine how good she felt about this!

The loss of weight and improvements in health changed these lives for the better in most cases. For example, one thirty-five-year-old man, Harry, had been a taxi driver, but when his weight increased to 370 pounds he no longer could fit behind the wheel of his cab. He lost his livelihood and his family went on public assistance. After surgery, his weight dropped to the low 200s. He went back to work in his taxi, but now had so much energy that he started to work a second shift as a dispatcher. This extra money helped him buy a house. I figured we saved the state of New York enough money on medical benefits to pay for all the other Medicaid patients I operated on that year.

Following their surgeries, some patients went back to school, others returned to the workforce or found better jobs now that they had more energy and a better appearance. One of my patients, Gloria, was a nurse in our hospital. I caught her pushing beds around only three weeks after her operation. Another patient, Ronald, was a "diet doctor" from North Carolina. He told me he was successful with everyone but himself. After the operation he told me he would take care of himself from then on, and returned home. I never saw him again, but apparently he did go back to his work soon after.

There are also some fairly bizarre stories. One of my very heaviest patients, Marilyn, weighed about 530 pounds. She had very large buttocks that extended out well behind her for several inches. This condition is called *steatopygia*. Her young grandchildren used to stand on this "shelf" and she would give them rides as she walked around the room. The inevitable happened when her postsurgery weight dropped to nearly 250 pounds. She lost her shelf, and the children complained about losing their rides. Not everyone was happy about the weight loss.

Actually, most of my patients were happy about their weight loss, even those who had some of the complications and problems from the operation. There were several studies by Solow, Silberforb, and Swift[2] and Brewer; White, and Baddeley[3] who compared patients before and after their intestinal-bypass operations. All of these studies reported an overall improvement of every aspect of psychological and social functioning. Anxiety and depression were decreased in most patients, and there was a much-improved mood. Physical activity and mobility were increased. They reported that such simple things as being able to cross their legs, sit comfortably in ordinary armchairs, sit in a movie theater, and pass through the checkout at supermarkets gave the patients great satisfaction. It was easier to buy clothing that was more stylish and colorful, and patients began to pay more attention to grooming and appearance. Their self-consciousness was decreased, and interpersonal relationships became more satisfying. Body image of surgery patients improved, as did their self-esteem. Sex was found to be more enjoyable, and there were a number of marriages and pregnancies. It is interesting that many of the patients became more self-assertive and outspoken. They stopped letting other people take advantage of them. Some stopped associating with obese friends, and tried to start a new life unrelated to their past. Of greatest importance was the fact that there was no tendency by these ex-morbidly obese individuals to substitute some other type of antisocial behavior for their former obesity. For most of them, overeating was no longer a compensation for all their problems.

There was a particularly strange comment that several patients made to me regarding their weight loss. It usually occurred after they lost at least 150 pounds. "Dr. Ackerman," they would say, "I have lost 150 pounds. That is a whole person. What's happened to that person?" Neither I nor the psychiatrist working with me knew how to answer such a question.

IMPROVEMENT IN DIABETES

The weight loss was only part of the success story that we saw in the early days of intestinal bypass. The most exciting changes in the health of the patients were the effects on diabetes and on serum cholesterol. Recall that many seriously obese patients had diabetes; they needed either daily insulin shots or pills to control the disease. We had even more patients who had slight to moderate increases in the amount of sugar in their blood, or whose blood sugars decreased abnormally slowly after drinking a sugary drink, in other words an abnormal glucose tolerance. While these latter groups of patients did not require any treatment, they were sometimes considered to be prediabetic or having chemical diabetes.

The relationship between excess weight and diabetes has been known for many years, and it has been shown that with the loss of weight many diabetics revert to a normal situation. So, as expected, after surgery, our diabetics got better. But the fact that the improvements occurred so early after surgery was unexpected. We studied a group of fifteen patients who had required either daily insulin injections or pills for control of their diabetes. Thirteen of them were able to discontinue completely their insulin or pills before discharge from the hospital, within ten days after the operation. Their blood sugar levels began to fall immediately after surgery, and there was even a noticeable decrease on the day after the operation. The two patients who still needed medicine for diabetes when discharged from the hospital were able to discontinue their insulin or pills completely during the next few weeks.

The blood sugar levels of virtually all of our patients became normal. In a few, the levels were still slightly elevated but did not require treatment. The glucose tolerance tests also improved, but this was a little strange. Even after drinking the sugary solution for the test, the blood sugar levels did not rise very much, almost as if the sugar was not completely absorbed into the bloodstream. This brought up the question of exactly why the diabetes improved.

There were probably several factors involved. The immediate improvements in blood sugar levels occurred before much weight was lost, so other factors besides weight reduction had to be involved. Weight loss undoubtedly was a factor many months later, and probably helped the patients to stay normal. But in the very early stages, the changes in diet were probably one of the important factors. In the hospital the patients didn't eat very much, and at home many spontaneously cut down on their caloric intake. This included a decrease in carbohydrate (a complex sugar) intake, and many patients expressed a loss of desire for excessive sweets. In addition, there was certainly evidence of a decrease in the absorption of carbohydrates, fats, and proteins that occurred after the operation. The patients became more responsive to the insulin that was produced by their bodies. This improvement in insulin sensitivity may have been due in part to changes in the production of certain polypeptide chemicals made by the intestine.

Whatever the factors, I am absolutely certain that weight loss itself was not important in these early stages. One of my patients conclusively proved this to me. Ida was a fifty-six-year-old woman who weighed about 400 pounds. As a diabetic she needed an injection of 60 units of insulin, a fairsized dose, every day. An intestinal bypass was performed, and her blood sugar levels started to decrease. Within a month after surgery they were normal, and she was able to stop her insulin injections. Weight loss was somewhat slow and she had some diarrhea. She became discouraged and decided that she wanted to be put back to "normal," even if it meant that her diabetes would return. I couldn't convince her otherwise, and reoperated on her, undoing the intestinal bypass. Reversing the surgery is a very straightforward operation. The connection of the functioning jejunum and ileum is separated, and the bypassed intestine is reattached to the functioning intestine, sewing the bypassed jejunum to the functioning jejunum and the bypassed ileum to the functioning ileum.

Immediately after the reversal, her blood sugar levels rose and within a brief period of time she had to resume her insulin injections. This occurred in spite of the fact that she tried to maintain her weight loss through dieting. In fact, her weight had been 378 pounds when I reversed the intestinal bypass, and four months later, with dieting, it was down further to 346 pounds. But her blood sugars were way up, very abnormal, and she was back on insulin injections. So clearly, there was something that happened when 90 percent of the intestine was bypassed that caused a decrease in blood sugars to the normal range, and this was unrelated to any weight loss!

I was very excited about this, and tried to find out more. I went back to my experimental laboratory and produced diabetes in a group of experimental animals (rats) with the use of a chemical called alloxan. This is a well-established technique that had been described a number of years ago. When I operated on and removed one-third of the upper part of the small intestine, the jejunum, the elevated blood sugars dropped to almost normal levels. The rats' water intake and urine output, which had been abnormal like that of a diabetic, returned to normal, and the glucose tolerance test became virtually normal. None of these changes occurred if the lower small intestine, the ileum, was removed. I was unable to proceed any further with this because of a lack of facilities and a basic lack of knowledge on my part of how to investigate further. (After all, I am not a diabetes doctor.) I published what I had done,[4] but nothing further has ever come out of it. This has been a big disappointment to me.

Finally, I should mention that the patients with slightly elevated blood sugar levels, and those with somewhat abnormal glucose tolerance tests all reached normal levels after the surgery.

IMPROVEMENTS IN SERUM LIPIDS

The other major improvement that occurred after the intestinal bypass involved cholesterol and triglycerides. Before the operation, twenty of our patients had very high levels of cholesterol in their blood (300–400 mg/dl), and twenty-five had elevated triglyceride levels. After the surgery, there was an average decrease of 50 percent in the cholesterol levels, and all of the patients reached normal levels. The greatest drop usually occurred within the first month after the operation. We continued this study for about two years, and the cholesterol levels remained normal (below 200 mg/dl or at least in the 200s) throughout this period. Our other patients who had normal cholesterol before surgery also experienced a 50 percent decrease in cholesterol.

The reasons for the improvements in cholesterol blood levels is interesting. First, obese patients seem to make more cholesterol in their bodies than thinner patients. Since not all obese people have high blood cholesterol levels, some of the cholesterol is passed out of the body in the bowel movements. Normally much of the cholesterol in the intestine is reabsorbed in the lower or small intestine (the ileum). When an intestinal bypass is performed, most of the ileum is bypassed, and a lot less of the intestinal cholesterol is absorbed. Instead, more of it passed out in the bowel movement, and the cholesterol levels in the blood fall. The body compensates for this lowering of cholesterol by producing more of it. But it can't keep up with the losses, and the levels stay lower. Another factor may be the decreased eating of fatty foods, which seems to occur spontaneously in some patients. Strangely enough, weight loss doesn't seem to be a very important factor, at least after intestinal bypasses.

Patients with abnormally elevated blood levels of triglycerides also had major improvements after intestinal bypass. These patients averaged a 65 percent drop in triglycerides, and all became normal. Even those whose triglyceride levels were normal before surgery had a fall in their blood levels, but to a much lesser extent. But the decrease in triglycerides was a very gradual one, and seemed to go down at a rate similar to the decrease in body weight. The major factors seem to be weight loss, and possibly changes in diet and physical activity.

There were other health benefits that occurred after the intestinal bypass, but they were all related to the weight loss itself and not to the fact that this particular operation was done. For the patients with high blood pressure, this meant that pressure was lowered, sometimes becoming completely normal. Patients who were taking medicine for their high blood pressure were able to discontinue the medication, or at least decrease the doses. I remember seeing one reported study by Solhaug and Bassoe[5] where average blood pressures in a group of patients dropped from 192/115, which is very high, to 146/88, close to normal, after weight loss from intestinal bypasses.

IMPROVEMENT IN RESPIRATORY STATUS

Similarly, breathing became easier for these morbidly obese patients after loss of a considerable amount of weight. Complaints about being short of breath after only minimal activity disappeared. The sophisticated breathing tests that were done all showed improvement in various functions of the lungs, including lung volume, distribution of gases within the lung, and the actual work involved in taking a breath. Our patients with the Pickwickian syndrome, a very serious problem involving the lungs, all became cured of this problem. The Pickwickian syndrome makes patients retain carbon dioxide in their bodies,which drives down the oxygen level. They may have trouble breathing and go into respiratory failure requiring mechanical support for their breathing. They may go into a coma, and death from respiratory or heart failure can occur. When excessive weight is lost, pulmonary function becomes normal and death is averted.

IMPROVEMENT IN ARTHRITIS

Improvement in back problems and arthritis of the weight-bearing joints was more variable. In those patients where complaints were due to constant strain because of the excess weight, changes were sometimes spectacular. Some who were almost bedridden before surgery were able to lead completely normal lives after the weight loss. But if damage to the joints before surgery had been extensive, even a very significant weight loss did not improve the situation all that much. Sometimes the arthritis was unrelated to the excess weight, as with patients suffering from rheumatoid arthritis, a serious form of arthritis unrelated to excess weight, and an autoimmune disease. Weight loss after the operation made life a little easier, but did not result in any major improvement of the arthritis.

Finally, some patients who needed joint-replacement surgery had been referred to me by orthopedic surgeons. The orthopedists felt that the joint replacement would fail because of the great amount of weight that would be put on the new joints. After the intestinal bypass, these patients lost enough weight to become reasonably good candidates for the joint-replacement operations. Several of these patients had total hip or total knee replacements with very good results. I remember one forty-one- year-old woman, Edna, who weighed about 215 pounds before her intestinal bypass. She had some congenital problems with her hips and legs, and was only 4 feet $7\frac{1}{2}$ inches tall. The arthritis in her hip joints was severe, and there had been two attempts to replace her hips. Both had failed. I should also mention that she had diabetes requiring daily insulin injections, and high cholesterol and triglyceride levels. She had a stormy course after her intestinal bypass, but eventually got better. About a year after her operation she underwent replacement of one hip, and then replacement of the other one. Both operations were successful. When I last saw her almost two years after the intestinal bypass, she weighed 123 pounds (a 43 percent weight loss), the diabetes was gone, and her cholesterol and triglycerides were normal. She was walking with a cane and was much improved.

Many of the patients were very happy with the results of the intestinal bypass, even if they developed some of the associated complications. Several said to me that they would rather die than have the operation reversed. What with the great weight loss and the improvements in all those medical problems it sounds very promising. But there were complications. The initial glowing reports of the patients' successes were quickly replaced by horror stories.

Overall, patients undergoing the intestinal bypass did well. The changes occurring in some of these patients were spectacular. Unfortunately for the patients and for the operation itself there were many complications. These encompassed many systems of the body and required intensive follow-up and very aggressive treatment. I personally learned a great deal about the human body from the troubles of these patients.

NOTES

1. C. S. W. Rand, J. M. Kuldau, and L. Robbins, "Surgery for Obesity and Marriage Quality," *JAMA* 247 (1982): 1419–22.

2. C. Solow, P. M. Silberfarb, and K. Swift, "Psychosocial Effects of Intestinal Bypass Surgery for Severe Obesity," *New England Journal of Medicine* 290 (1974): 300–304.

3. C. Brewer, H. White, and M. Baddeley, "Beneficial Effects of Jejunoileostomy on Compulsive Eating and Associated Psychiatric Symptoms," *British Medical Journal* 4 (1974): 314–16.

4. N. B. Ackerman, "Experimental Studies on the Control of Diabetes Mellitus by Jejunal Exclusion," *Langenbecks Archiv fuer Chirurgie* 357 (1982): 171.

5. J. H. Solhaug and H. H. Bassoe, "Jejuno-Ileal Bypass Operations for the Treatment of Morbid Obesity," *Scandinavian Journal of Gastroenterology* 14 (1979): 535–43.

13

Complications of Intestinal Bypass

Those naturally fat are more liable to sudden death than the thin.
—Hippocrates, *Aphorisms*

The intestinal bypass looked like a good operation to those of us involved with it, but more and more complications began to be reported. Fortunately we do have a better type of operation for morbid obesity—the gastric bypass. It cannot be denied that many of morbidly obese people were helped by the intestinal bypass.

DIARRHEA

We already knew about the diarrhea. This started a few days after the surgery when intestinal function began. Just about every patient had diarrhea. Its intensity and extent varied from a relatively mild problem of three to four bowel movements per day, fully controlled, to a very intensive diarrhea of twenty to thirty bowel movements per day.

There seemed to be several causes of the diarrhea. First, transit time, the time it took for movement of gastrointestinal contents from top to bottom was more rapid. We would see this if we ordered an X-ray of the abdomen after giving the patient barium to swallow. The barium, which shows up on X-ray, moved down through the intestinal tract with record speed. Also, because of the surgically shortened intestine, there was a lot less surface area to absorb the fluid in the intestine, and the bowel movements remained liquid. Certain substances in the intestinal fluid that were not absorbed well added to the irritation of the intestine. These included bile salts from the liver, and fatty acids. If all this weren't enough, there were some other factors involved. Overeating, drinking large quantities of fluid, eating certain foods, and emotional problems all added to the difficulties with the diarrhea. Cold, icy liquids were particularly troublesome. It sometimes helped if patients drank their liquids between meals rather than with their food.

The relationship between emotional problems and diarrhea was an interesting one. Some patients noted that while they were working, or otherwise distracted the diarrhea was less severe. For some, evenings and weekends at home were particularly bad. I remember one patient, Rose, whose diarrhea was so bad that she had to be hospitalized to try to control it. As soon as she entered the hospital the diarrhea stopped. When she went home it started. This happened several times. I had a long talk with her to try to make her realize what was happening. Something was going on at home to irritate her, in every sense of the word. I never found out exactly what it was, but she eventually learned to cope with the problems and the diarrhea lessened.

Fortunately, for many patients there was a tendency for the diarrhea to decrease with time. Many patients ultimately needed no medication to control it. But there were many instances when the diarrhea flared up again, sometimes more than a year after the operation.

The diarrhea—ten to twenty loose bowel movements per day—is bad enough but the diarrhea caused all sorts of other problems. Some were just irritating and uncomfortable, but some were potentially dangerous. First of all, the diarrhea was often very irritating, and sometimes causing pain to the anal area. Some patients needed narcotic pain medicine to give them relief until we could get the diarrhea under control. At times, hemorrhoids, fissures (cracks in the skin), or severe inflammation occurred. I had a battery of ointments and suppositories to prescribe, and these usually helped.

More serious than this were the problems that resulted from deficiencies of potassium, calcium, and magnesium. These deficiencies occurred in patients who had severe diarrhea, but there were other factors involved, like decreased intestinal absorption as a result of the operation, changes in diet, and vomiting. Potassium deficiency caused muscle weakness and pain, poor coordination, dizziness, loss of appetite, and many other problems. Patients with this problem sometimes needed hospitalization and urgent replacement of the potassium. Magnesium deficiency caused similar problems as well as mental changes and confusion. Calcium deficiency was even more complicated. Calcium deficiency caused muscle cramps and spasms, which were sometimes very serious. In addition to all the other reasons for its occurrence, poor absorption of Vitamin D also seemed to play a role in the calcium deficiency. Exceptionally large doses of this vitamin were frequently given to treat these patients, as well as very high doses of calcium.

KIDNEY STONES

Some patients experienced kidney stones, or calcium oxalate stones to be more specific. Normally, oxalate, which is present in many of the foods we eat, combines with calcium in the intestines and is passed out in the bowel movement without causing any problems. But patients with an intestinal bypass have an increased amount of fat in the large intestine because fat is not absorbed normally. The calcium in the intestine combines with this fat rather than with the oxalate. Instead, the oxalate gets absorbed in the bloodstream, and it eventually gets to the kidneys where it combines there with calcium to form stones or crystals. These unfortunate patients may develop severe pain from the stones, and some eventually get destruction of the kidneys with loss of function. Obviously this is extremely serious. We tried to avoid kidney problems by giving high doses of calcium, and by putting patients on a low-oxalate diet. The problem was that many foods contain oxalates. These included many vegetables such as spinach, green beans, beets, chard, rhubarb, endive, and okra; fruits such as berries, grapes, figs, currents, plums, and citrus fruits; and almonds, cashew nuts, chocolate, tea, and coffee.

LIVER DAMAGE

Possibly the most serious problem potentially facing the intestinal-bypass patient was liver damage. Fortunately the incidence of this was fairly low, but when it occurred it was often life threatening. It appeared to be related to protein malnutrition, especially occurring during the period of greatest weight loss. It was similar to a disease of protein malnutrition that occurs in Third World countries called *Kwashiorkor*. Patients of mine with these liver problems either had an increased loss of protein because of very excessive diarrhea, or were getting less protein into their digestive tract because of vomiting or changes in diet, or a combination of these factors. One patient told me that she had moved, and the stove in the new house had not been connected for many weeks. She had stopped eating a well-rounded, protein-containing diet, and developed early signs of liver failure. Another patient started to drink alcoholic beverages because of worsening family problems; his diarrhea increased as his food intake decreased. In all of these patients, blood levels of albumin (a type of protein found in the blood) and protein decreased. We found that by giving appropriate oral or intravenous protein-containing fluids to these patients we could reverse any damage to the liver and get them back to a normal condition. One of my patients had liver problems develop three times during the first two years after surgery. She needed three intensive courses of protein-replacement treatment, until finally the liver problems disappeared. A number of surgeons reported that some patients had progressed from liver failure to coma and death when irreversible liver changes developed before protein replacement was started.

ARTHRALGIA

Another annoying, but not life-threatening problem that sometimes develops is arthritis, or to be more accurate, arthralgia. Arthralgia means painful joints, rather than the inflamed, damaged joints of arthritis. This could occur within a few weeks after the operation or several years later. The symptoms include morning stiffness and involvement of many joints. Joint involvement is not necessarily the same on both sides of the body. The joints are painful, reddened, and often swollen, and symptoms may involve the neck, elbows, back, ankles, knees, shoulders, wrists, and fingers. These symptoms last for a few days or for several weeks, and sometimes return after a period when the joints have been completely normal. In some patients the problems totally disappear without returning. It is believed that the arthralgia is related to antigens (substances that stimulate production of antibodies) from certain bacteria in the bypassed intestine. Treatment with aspirin and other anti-inflammatory drugs is usually successful, but some patients need stronger medications, such as cortisone or prednisone (adrenal hormones used to treat inflammation).

I had one patient, Lily, who developed arthritis about four months after her intestinal bypass. The rheumatologists felt that this was probably not "bypass arthritis," since the tests for rheumatoid arthritis were positive. But some doubts about the diagnosis persisted. Since "bypass arthritis" totally disappears when the intestinal bypass is reversed, it was agreed that this should be done. I performed the surgery, converting the intestinal bypass to a gastric bypass. Her excellent 46 percent weight loss was retained, but unfortunately the arthritis did not disappear. It was, indeed, rheumatoid arthritis, unrelated to the intestinal bypass.

There are a number of other complications that can confront the patient at any time after the intestinal bypass. I think you can begin to see why the enthusiasm for this operation started to diminish.

GASTROINTESTINAL-TRACT PROBLEMS

Some of these complications directly involved the gastrointestinal tract. Some patients suffer from nausea and vomiting almost immediately after the operation. For some, this is relatively mild and shortlived. For others it is more of a problem. Sometimes it is hard to find out why the patient has the nausea and vomiting. Occasionally it is related to some medicine we give. At other times we have the feeling that it is some kind of emotional response to the surgery. One doctor, skilled at hypnosis, tried to stop the vomiting with hypnotic suggestion. Surprisingly, this worked in possibly half of our vomiters. I remember one patient who had only one session with the hypnotist, who told the patient that the nausea and vomiting would stop as soon as she awakened. It did! Vomiting is potentially a very serious problem for these patients. Remember, they are also having diarrhea at the same time. So they are losing fluids, minerals, and proteins quite rapidly, and not replacing them fast enough. In addition, these patients are not absorbing what little fluid, vitamins, and minerals they do hold down. These are the patients who can develop liver failure, severe dehydration, and mineral depletion unless the vomiting and diarrhea are successfully managed. Frequently they are rehospitalized so we can work on them to get these problems under control.

Many intestinal-bypass patients suffer from excessive gas and cramps in their intestines. Sometimes this is exceedingly uncomfortable, and although relieved by passing the gas, the odors produced are foul smelling. This is believed to be due to the overgrowth of bacteria in the bypassed part of the intestine. Often this problem clears up by itself, but it is fairly difficult to treat when persistent.

Other more serious gastrointestinal complications are fortunately much less common. Obstruction can occur at various locations in the intestines. The diagnosis of this is sometimes very difficult. X-rays of an obstructed intestine usually show certain patterns of intestinal gas that help pin down the diagnosis. But the intestinal-bypass patients always have a large amount of gas in the intestine, and this mimicks the obstructed pattern even when obstruction is not present. Sometimes obstruction is due to a twisting of the intestine or to an accordion-like collapsing of the intestine into itself. Usually an exploratory operation is necessary to diagnose and relieve the obstruction.

There is also a condition known as "bypass enteritis" in which patients have a sudden increase in diarrhea, abdominal pain, nausea, and a high temperature, all of which imply an acute inflammation of the intestine. It is hard to diagnose, and in fact is probably greatly overdiagnosed. We have never really been able to find out why this occurs and what brings it on.

OTHER PROBLEMS

Many other problems plague these bypass patients. Some are relatively common, such as temporary hair loss. Researchers are not absolutely sure why there is hair loss in some of these patients. Deficiencies in such things as protein, vitamins, and zinc have been suggested, but nothing has been substantiated. This not only occurs in some intestinal-bypass patients, but also can occur in anyone who has a major weight loss, for any reason, including dieting. Hair loss is minimal, and spontaneously grows back within a few weeks to a few months. But patients, particularly the women, can get very panicked about it until they are reassured that this hair will all grow back. Often I hear them say, "This is some operation! I'm going to be a skinny bald woman!" But it does grow back.

Some patients complain of coldness, even during the warmest parts of the year. It was believed to be due to a reduction of the fatty layer of insulation just beneath the skin. These chills are also felt after other methods of weight loss. I have had patients who tell me they are putting on sweaters in the heat of the summer while everyone else is taking them off.

More serious, but fortunately much more uncommon are such problems as tuberculosis in other areas of the body than the lungs, pancreatic inflammation, and an unusual form of encephalopathy.

Although most patients experience positive emotional benefits from the intestinal bypass, there are some negative results. There have been a few reports of depression occurring after the operation, occasionally followed by some suicides. With the help of psychiatry, appropriate medicines, and time, most of the emotional stress improves.

DEATHS

Finally, there are deaths directly and indirectly due to the operation and its aftermath. Most of the deaths do not happen right after the operation, but occur much later. The most common causes are severe dehydration and mineral depletion, alcoholism and liver failure, the sudden death syndrome, kidney failure, pancreatic inflammatory disease, tuberculosis, and intestinal complications. Probably about 2 to 4 percent of intestinal-bypass patients die from these problems.

Weight loss from intestinal bypass is generally excellent, but the complications are often serious and disabling. Fortunately many of the complications can be treated successfully, and if all else fails, the operation can be reversed. Unfortunately, "All else does fail" in a fairly high percentage of patients. I used to say that 50 percent needed reversing, 25 percent were having major problems but were coping with them, and 25 percent were doing well. But now I just don't know. If the operation is reversed most patients gradually gain back all of the lost weight, often virtually to the exact pound. But that's where the gastric bypass comes in. If the intestinal bypass is reversed and a gastric bypass is done at the same time, the weight loss is usually maintained.

14

What About Other Operations?

He who distinguishes the true savor of his food can never be a glutton;
he who does not cannot be otherwise.

—Henry David Thoreau

Surgeons tend to be innovative. Every surgeon has his or her own way of conducting an operation that may be slightly, or not so slightly, different than anyone else's way of doing the same operation. Surgeons tend to invent new operations or variations on older ones, and many of these new operations are based on good, sound medical principles. (And some are not.) The same can be said of surgical approaches to severe obesity. Before we get into the gastric bypass and the gastric restrictive operations, we should mention some of the other operations that have been suggested, including some that have absolutely failed.

There have been a number of variations proposed for improving the results of the intestinal bypass. Some of this we have already discussed, such as whether to use an end-to-end or an end-to-side connection (see Fig. 5, p. 50). One of the earliest types of intestinal bypass was the jejuno-colostomy (see Fig. 4, p. 49), where the shortened upper small intestine, the jejunum, was connected directly to the colon, or large intestine. This operation was discarded in the early days of intestinal bypasses because of totally unpredictable weight loss and a very high rate of complications. But there were other interesting suggestions.

Treatment for Inadequate Weight Loss

Some patients with an intestinal bypass did not lose enough weight after the operation, or started to regain weight after having lost a significant number of pounds. In my experience this occurs in less than 10 percent of patients. But what can be done for these few unfortunate people? There are two possibilities. The first is to reoperate and shorten further the amount of functioning small intestine. When we reoperate on these patients, we find that the functioning intestine "compensates" for the shortening by widening its diameter, thickening its lining, and increasing its length. By actual measurement we find that the length increased by more than 50 percent. The result is much more surface area and absorption of calories and nutrients increased. So we do the obvious. We remove some of the lengthened part of the intestine, usually about 40 percent by measurement. This procedure works pretty well, and most patients lose more weight, dropping to an average loss of 35 percent of their starting weight. Well, this has no beneficial effect on the complication rate, and sometimes more complications result. So the ultimate answer is to undo the intestinal bypass and perform a gastric bypass.

Treatment for the Complications

There are also two possible ways of managing the patient who has serious complications from the intestinal bypass. Since many of the complications are related to the very short length of functioning small intestine, an obvious approach is to try to lengthen this part of the intestine. There are several ways to do this, but they usually involve adding about 8 to 14 inches of functioning intestine. I did this for three patients, and they fared pretty well without any real weight gain. But again, the ultimate answer turns out to be its reversal and a conversion to a gastric bypass.

Duodenoileal Bypass

More innovative than all of this are the attempts to salvage the intestinal-bypass operation by making some basic changes in what gets connected to what. In one operation for example, the surgeons connect the very beginning of the jejunum, just beyond the duodenum (the first part of the small intestine) to the ileum, bypassing virtually all of the jejunum and only part of the ileum. In this operation, called the *duodenoileal bypass*, the idea is to have the functioning part of the intestine include a relatively large length of ileum. Supposedly the patients develop fewer complications after this operation. But the operation never became popular. It belongs to medical history now. Interest has turned toward the stomach and the gastric-bypass operations rather than any variations of the intestinal bypass for treatment of morbid obesity.

BILIOINTESTINAL BYPASS

An operation that I view as more innovative is the *biliointestinal bypass*. In this variation of the intestinal bypass the gallbladder is directly connected to the bypassed part of the intestine. Remember, about 90 percent of the small intestine is bypassed. With this new operation, almost all of the bile from the gallbladder is absorbed in this long segment of the intestine, and as a result bouts of diarrhea are less severe. Of course, if the patient has gallbladder disease or if it had previously been removed, this new operation is impossible. This interesting operation has not "caught on." It too belongs to medical history.

When the complications from the intestinal bypass become too overwhelming, something has to be done. Simply reoperating and undoing or taking down the intestinal bypass is not the definitive answer. The complications might go away, but the patients start to gain back all their lost weight. It is gradual, but usually goes on and on until reaching essentially the preoperative level, sometimes to the exact pound. So something else has to be done to protect the weight loss. That something is the gastric bypass. This is done preferably at the same time as the reversal of the intestinal bypass. I have done this combined procedure as early as six months after the original intestinal bypass, and as late as seventeen years later. Most of the patients did not gain weight after this combined operation, and most of the other benefits persist. In particular, blood sugar levels in former diabetics remain normal, as do blood levels of triglycerides. The only exception is that the blood cholesterol levels rise nearly to preoperative values. I guess nothing is perfect. But overall, the conversion to a gastric bypass has been very satisfactory.

There is very little else to say about the intestinal bypass. I think there may still be a few surgeons performing these operations occasionally, but for the most part stomach-stapling operations have taken over.

PLASTIC SURGERY

There are still a few other surgical procedures to discuss. The plastic surgeons have a lot of skills that are helpful in treating the very obese patient.
But remember that most morbidly obese people have excessive fat
deposits throughout their bodies—abdomens, thighs, buttocks, hips,
arms, and so on. There is no way that any surgeon, even a plastic surgeon,
can remove all the fat in all these areas. What I'm getting at is that the
plastic surgical operations are useful in removing fat and excess skin in
local areas of the body. They are particularly good for some patients who
have lost a lot of weight but still have excess, sagging skin. We'll discuss
in chapter 23 the value of plastic surgery in our postoperative patients.

You might raise some questions about what I've just written. How
about the patient who has a very large, sagging, fat abdominal wall, like
an exaggerated "beer belly"? Wouldn't he or she benefit from the surgical removal of the skin and underlying fat of this area? Well, it all
depends. If the skin and fat are so excessive that they hang down to the
thighs or even knees, removal may have some value. The skin gets very
heavy, may be very difficult to keep clean, especially underneath where it
rubs on the skin below it, and infections can develop. The problem with
the surgery, which is called a *panniculectomy* or an *abdominoplasty*, is
that a very large area of fatty tissue is exposed after the skin is cut off, and
when this is sewn back together again a massive infection can develop. I
remember seeing a patient who did develop such an infection, and the
patient almost died. This type of operation is really best when it is done
on a patient who has lost a lot of weight and has excess skin but not much
underlying fat. More about this in chapter 23.

JAW WIRING

I think one of the most interesting operations is the wiring of the jaws to
prevent the patient from overeating. The principle is obvious. With the
jaws wired closed the patient can take in only a liquid diet with restricted
calories. It does result in a major change in one's daily life, and candidates
for this must be emotionally prepared for it. Also a relatively healthy set
of teeth is a necessity. This is a dental procedure performed by oral surgeons. There apparently are several ways to do this. Usually it is done with
heavy wires, but there is also a method that uses heavy elastic bands.

Patients with wired jaws are put on a liquid diet. One such 800-calorie diet consists of milk, tomato juice, fruit juice, and vitamins. Another diet, also 800 calories, consists of fluids and liquefied soft food such as soft-boiled eggs. Some patients complain of mild discomforts such as dry lips, soreness of the gums, and bad breath. There is one potentially serious problem that can occur. If the patient has to vomit, for any reason, there is the possibility that the vomited material may get into the patient's airway and interfere with breathing. I have read of one such case in which the patient actually suffered a cardiac arrest. For this reason, the patients are sometimes given a pair of wire cutters to be used in an emergency.

Jaw wiring is not used as a lifelong method for weight loss. I don't think anyone could put up with this for a very long period of time. Usually the jaws are wired for about six months, but there is considerable variation for individual cases. Sometimes the wires are removed for a while and then reinserted. Some patients have had jaws wired for as long as twelve months. But eventually the wires are discontinued. The problem is that while weight loss is fairly good at first, a leveling off usually occurs. The patients may lose fifty or sixty pounds, which is quite impressive. But when the wires are removed, most patients start to regain their weight gradually. Some regain all of the weight they lost. All of this is similar to what happens to most patients after they stop dieting. What is needed is some way to keep this lost weight off, for a long period. The best suggestion has been to use jaw wiring as a preliminary procedure in treating the very heaviest morbidly obese patients. Then when the wires are removed, the patient should immediately undergo a gastric-stapling operation. I have never had the opportunity to do this, but I think it is a good idea.

Jaw wiring does not always work. I had one patient who had her jaws wired with the heavy elastic bands. She told me that she was able to pry her jaws apart just enough to get a forkful of food into her mouth. She figured that she had the best of all possible worlds, jaws wired for weight loss and the ability to eat what she wanted. Of course she lost no weight at all. The lesson is, if there is a way to cheat, most morbidly obese patients will find it.

HYPOTHALAMIC TREATMENT

The next procedure to discuss is really innovative, and is based on classic scientific research. It has been known for many years that part of the brain, the hypothalamus, is involved in the regulation of food intake. If it is injured in one area increased food intake and obesity can result. But injuries to another nearby area of the same part of the brain lead to the opposite, decreased eating and loss of weight. Most of this knowledge came from experimental work on animals such as rats and mice dating back to the 1940s and 1950s. There have been patients who have had brain injuries or tumors in these areas that have resulted in changes in eating habits, particularly the development of obesity.

I am aware of one attempt to use this knowledge in the treatment of a group of morbidly obese patients. This was in Denmark by Quaade, Vernet, and Larsson,[1] and involved operating on five very obese people. They were, of course, told that this was experimental, and gave their consent. The neurosurgeon first electrically stimulated the area of the hypothalamus that causes increased appetite, and three of the five patients reported a sudden, intense hunger. In these three patients the stimulated area was then burnt by an electrical current. One patient had this done on both sides of the brain.

Unfortunately the results of the experiment have not been great. The three treated patients all said it took less food to give them the feeling of fullness, and they decreased their intake of food to some degree. But actual weight loss did not occur, and all effects lasted for only a short period of time. It's still a fascinating idea, but nothing practical has yet resulted.

BILIOPANCREATIC BYPASS

The final operation to be discussed is the *biliopancreatic bypass*. This is the one operation that I have never totally understood. It was devised by a very clever Italian surgeon, Dr. Nicola Scopinaro. The operation is meant to improve upon the intestinal bypass by eliminating some of its problems, particularly the diarrhea. It is a major operation in which the gastrointestinal tract is rearranged so that there are three parts, all connected to each other (Fig. 6). These three parts are: the upper half of the small intestine including the area that receives the bile from the liver, the lower part of the small intestine which the surgeon connects to the stomach, and the very lowest part of the small intestine which is connected to both of the above. With this operation the bile is absorbed in a normal fashion, but it is diverted away from the stomach. This is good because

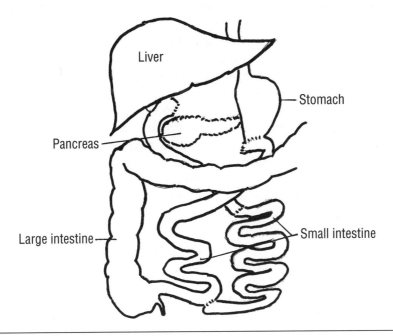

Fig. 6. Biliopancreatic bypass

the diarrhea is decreased, but potentially bad because stomach ulcers could develop when the bile is diverted so far away from the stomach. So an additional part of the operation involves the removal of the lower half of the stomach to prevent ulcers.

Supposedly, the biliopancreatic bypass provides a selective decrease in the absorption of fats and starches, but absorption of sugars and proteins is relatively unaffected. I'm not sure I completely understand this. But the results do seem fairly good. Bouts of diarrhea are minimal and weight loss seems satisfactory. After this operation, there is a potential for the formation of kidney stones and also of gallstones. Frankly, it seems to be a very big operation, with a lot of intestinal suturing and a major removal of half of the stomach. I'm not sure that an operation of this magnitude is justified or necessary. I believe the operation is still being done by surgeons in several places in the United States and Europe. We will have to see how research here progresses.

I did have one experience with this operation, or at least with a patient who had had it done by a surgeon in California. The patient came to me because she had developed a rare neurological condition after she had the biliopancreatic bypass. She was experiencing weakness and pain in her legs, and a tingling sensation in her arms. On some days she had difficulty even getting out of bed. Her doctors weren't sure that this was directly related to the bypass operation, but they wondered if the condition would disappear if the bypassed was reversed. I wasn't sure either. The patient had lost a fair amount of weight, about 88 pounds, and didn't want to gain it back. After extensive discussions, we decided to reverse the biliopancreatic bypass and replace it with a gastric bypass at the same operation. This was complicated. I had never operated on anyone who previously had a biliopancreatic bypass. Before the reversal surgery, I drew a lot of diagrams, and finally worked out what I would do. It was so complicated that I actually took my final drawing into the operating room with me so that I could refer to it during the operation. I have never done that before. My diagram listed seven steps to be performed, and there were six suture lines involving the intestine and stomach. It worked out well. After the operation, the patient kept her weight off, actually losing some additional weight. Happily, the neurological problems completely disappeared.

These other operations are all very interesting, although of very little practical value. They demonstrate very clearly the innovative side of surgeons. However, the complete change of direction represented by the emergence of the gastric bypass as the therapy for morbid obesity is really remarkable. This is presented in great detail in the next chapter.

NOTE

1. F. Quaade, K. Vernet, and S. Larsson, "Stereotaxic Stimulation and Electrocoagulation of the Lateral Hypothalamus in Obese Humans," *Acta Neurochirurgica* 30 (1974): 111–17.

15

The Emergence of Stomach Stapling

The fool that eats till he is sick must fast till he is well.
—George Walter Thornbury, *The Jestor's Sermon*

While many surgeons, including me, were busy doing the intestinal bypass to treat our morbidly obese patients, another very different type of operation was being developed, this time involving the stomach rather than the intestine. I've been referring to it as the gastric bypass or the stomach-stapling operation, but technically speaking, that's not completely correct. There are several basic principles in these operations, but there are many ways to accomplish them. In other words, there are many variations of the basic surgery.

PRINCIPLES

The first basic principle is to make the part of the stomach that receives the food very small, so that the patient will eat much less. This can be done with special stainless staples, or it can be done with stitches. Thus not all these operations involve stapling, although most surgeons now do use the staples.

The second basic principle is to make the outlet of this small stomach very narrow, so that emptying of the food from the stomach will be delayed. By this means, the patient feels full for many hours, and the desire, or even the ability to eat between meals is drastically reduced, or

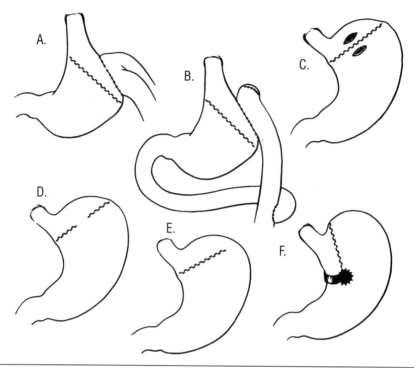

Fig. 7. Gastric operations: (a) loop gastric bypass, (b) Roux-en-Y gastric bypass, (c) gastrogastrostomy, (d) and (e) gastroplasties, and (f) vertical banded gastroplasty. (Reprinted by permission, *Gastrointestinal Surgery* 2 [1985])

even eliminated. This can be accomplished with stitches, staples, or various plastic or metal bands.

In the true gastric-bypass operation, the food goes directly from the small, upper part of the stomach, or gastric pouch as I call it, to the intestine, through an opening made between the two organs. In these operations, the lower part of the stomach, which includes most of the stomach, is bypassed. Hence the name gastric bypass. But there are other ways to accomplish the two basic principles (Fig. 7). Instead, the upper gastric pouch can be made to empty directly through a narrow opening into the lower part of the stomach. In these operations the stomach is not bypassed, so another name is needed. Well, these operations are called *gastroplasties*. The suffix "plasty" is from the Greek, and means to form, mold, or shape.

The whole group of stomach-related operations—gastric bypass, gastric stapling, and gastroplasty—really only refer to specific techniques. Some people use the term *gastric restrictive procedures* to refer to them. It is accurate but it seems a bit clumsy. For convenience sake I'm going to use the term *gastric bypass* for the whole group of operations, but I'll use the specific name whenever I talk about a specific operation.

HISTORY OF DEVELOPMENT

Now for a little history. In the mid-1960s when many surgeons were beginning to do the intestinal bypass on morbidly obese patients, the idea of a gastric bypass was just starting to be developed.

The developer of the gastric-bypass procedures was Dr. Edward Mason, who had taken his surgery-residency training at the University of Minnesota about ten years before I had. In the mid-1940s at Minnesota there was a lot of interest in the surgery of patients who had stomach and duodenal ulcers. The prevailing operation at that time was the *Billroth II gastrectomy*. Theodor Billroth was probably the greatest Viennese surgeon of the late 1800s. He devised several operations for ulcers, the Billroth II being the second one. In this operation much of the stomach was removed, and the upper part remaining was then connected to the jejunum. The operation was an effective one with elimination of ulcers in all but a few patients. But because the remaining part of the stomach was sometimes made fairly small, many patients had difficulty regaining any lost weight.

Mason completed his surgical residency training and moved to the University of Iowa. In 1966 to 1970, he performed his first gastric-bypass operations on morbidly obese patients. He was not sure how small the gastric pouch had to be, and he made the connection between the stomach and intestine fairly large, about 2 centimeters wide. The pouch sometimes stretched and increased in size, and the connection, called the *stoma*, also occasionally stretched. In spite of this, most of his patients experienced considerable weight loss.

This operation was controversial, and was condemned by some surgeons. When the lower half of the stomach, the *antrum*, is separated from the upper half of the stomach, the *fundus*, ulcers can develop. Bile from the intestine can back up into the antrum and cause the release by the antrum of a chemical called *gastrin*. Gastrin then causes the secretion of increased amounts of hydrochloric acid from the fundus and ulcers can result. Fortunately, this does not occur with a gastric bypass. The reason is that the antrum and the fundus are not really separated. The gastric pouch is made so small that most of the fundus is still connected with the antrum beyond the limits of the gastric pouch. So if gastrin is produced by the antrum, the acid from the fundus runs into the antrum, neutralizes the bile, and stops the release of gastrin.

Well, it took a while before Mason and his colleagues at Iowa convinced everyone of this, showing them that the gastric-bypass patients rarely develop problems with ulcers. After this, the popularity of gastric bypass began to rise.

In 1971, Mason changed direction and devised the first *gastroplasty*. He divided the stomach as he did with his gastric bypasses, but left a small part of the stomach on the left side undivided, still intact, similar to Fig. 7E (p. 114). This was now his stoma or connection between the upper pouch and the rest of the stomach. But again, the pouch was too big and the stoma too wide. He stopped doing these gastroplasties and returned to the gastric bypass for the rest of the 1970s.

Mason continued to try to improve the operation during this time. A major change occurred in 1976 when Dr. John Alden, a surgeon in St. Paul, Minnesota, started using surgical staples to separate the upper pouch from the rest of the stomach. In Mason's operations the stomach was actually cut and divided, which made the pouch and lower stomach completely separate. Alden felt, correctly, that the stomach only needed to be partitioned so that no food would enter the lower stomach, and that this partitioning could effectively be done with staples (see Fig. 7A). These small stainless-steel staples had been used for other types of stomach and intestinal surgery, and were tolerated well by the body. The instrument that he used placed thirty-three staples in two parallel rows completely across the upper part of the stomach. This technique simplified the operation, and was adopted by many, including Mason.

The next major development occurred at about the same time. In the gastric-bypass operation, the stomach was connected to a "loop" of small intestine. That is to say, the pulling up of the intestine to join with the stomach makes the intestine appear in the shape of a loop. This was, and is perfectly all right, but some patients were having problems relating to the loop and to bile. The bile, flowing from the liver to the intestine, passed inside the intestine in a normal fashion without problems until it reached the area of the stomach. Then, in some patients, the bile went through the stoma connecting the intestine and the stomach. Bile can be very irritating, and in these patients an inflammation of the stomach and esophagus occurred.

To avoid this problem, many surgeons stopped using a loop of intestine, and switched to what is called a "Roux-en-Y" (pronounced roo-en-why). This procedure, named after the Swiss surgeon Cesar Roux (see Fig. 7B), divides the loop close to the place where the intestine is connected to the stomach, and then connects this divided part to the intestine way beyond the stomach. This way, the bile never gets up to the stomach, and the irritation is prevented. It does make the operation a little more complicated, and adds more lines of suturing. Some surgeons, including me, rarely have a problem with the bile, and continue to use the loop technique (see Fig. 7A). By the way, the connection of this part of the intestine, the jejunum, to a part of the jejunum beyond the stomach is called a "jejunojejunostomy."

The surgical pendulum began to swing again, and variations on the gastroplasty principle started to gain popularity. The pouch size was greatly reduced. Staples were used to partition the stomach, but a gap in the row of staples could be used to create a stoma between the pouch and the lower stomach. With this as the basic technique, variations started to appear. Some surgeons made the gap, or stoma on the left side of the stomach, the so-called greater curvature of the stomach (see Fig. 7E). Others made the stoma on the right side, the lesser curvature of the stomach. The only remaining possibility was to use the central portion of the stomach as the stoma (see Fig. 7D), and sure enough, this was also tried. This third option was accomplished by placing staples all across the stomach except for the area that was to be the stoma in the central part. Other variations included putting the staples horizontally across the stomach or vertically up to the esophagus.

One other interesting variation was the *gastrogastrostomy* (see Fig. 7C). This involved stapling totally across the stomach, horizontally, and then making two small openings in the stomach, one above and one below the staple line. Then these two small openings were sewn together, creating a stoma that connected the small upper stomach pouch with the lower stomach.

FINE TUNING

After all these variations were developed, the fine tuning of gastric bypasses and gastroplasties began. There were a number of basic questions to be answered. How big should the gastric pouch be? How narrow should the stoma be? How can we protect the staple line from separating and pulling apart? How can we prevent the stoma from stretching?

Every physician had his or her own ideas on these questions. Every year we await the announcement of the new "operation of the year." The stomach pouches are made smaller and smaller. One surgeon told me that he did not make a pouch, but instead made a "passageway" for the food to progress from the esophagus to the intestine. Elaborate methods were devised to measure the size of the pouch accurately. Some surgeons hit upon making the pouches 20 cubic centimeters in size, about two-thirds of an ounce. Others made their pouches capable of holding one to two ounces.

The width of the stoma also varied. Most surgeons created openings from about 5 millimeters to 12 millimeters in width, with 8 to 10 mm probably being the most popular. But one surgeon made his gastric and intestinal openings only 3 millimeters wide, and then wondered why some of his patients became obstructed at the site of the stoma.

How to prevent the line of staples from pulling apart or disrupting was an important problem. As we'll discuss later, disruption of the staples was, and possibly still is, one of the major causes of failures of the operations. Let me explain how this stapling is done. The stainless-steel staples come packaged in a small cartridge that fits into the stapling instrument. The instrument is positioned across the stomach, tightened up, and then "fired." A total of thirty-three small staples become imbedded in the wall of the stomach, in two close parallel rows. One would think this would be strong enough, but it isn't, and opening up of the staple line can occur. Some surgeons have added a row of nonabsorbable stitches beyond the staples. Others have fired a second cartridge of thirty-three more staples, beyond the first rows. I even know of a surgeon who placed a *third* row of thirty-three more staples. What appears to have worked best is a new instrument that fires sixty-six staples in four close parallel rows. Somehow this instrument, the TA-90B made by the U.S. Surgical Company, seems to work better than using two cartridges of thirty-three staples each. Possibly it's the spacing of the four rows that accounts for the greater success.

Finally, it is important to protect the stoma from stretching or dilating. I think normally some stretching does occur. There was one study where the surgeons looked into the stomach, using endoscopes, in patients shortly after their gastric bypasses, and at three-month intervals. An *endoscope* is an instrument that is passed down through the mouth into the stomach, and with the help of its light source and lens, permits the endoscopist to look into the interior of the stomach. After the operation, the stoma's size averaged 9 mm or 0.35 inches wide. A year later, the average size was 17 mm or 0.67 inches. But the patients had good results in terms of weight loss, so some stretching is acceptable. But when the stomas stretch to 25 to 30 mm or more or 0.98 to 1.18 inches, there is a real problem. I have even measured a stoma that stretched all the way up to 66 mm or 2.6 inches in width. How to prevent this from happening? If the stoma stretches too much, food could empty from the stomach too rapidly. I think this still is an unsolved question. Surgeons have reinforced the stomas with various types of stitches at the borders. Others have used plastic rings or bands around the stomas, or even metal rings. These techniques have not been uniformly successful. In fact, sometimes the plastic or metal works its way into the wall of the stomach, eventually getting inside the stomach. The stomach seals itself off as this gradually occurs, so that there is no perforation occurring. But once inside the stomach, the plastic or metal can obstruct the stoma and cause bleeding from the stomach lining. Sometimes the patient may even have to be reoperated on as a result. So we are still looking for a good answer for this problem.

OTHER GASTRIC OPERATIONS

The inventiveness of the surgical mind has not yet reached its limits. Let me tell you about *gastric wrapping* and *gastric banding*.

Gastric wrapping is the more radical of these operations. It is argued that the capacity of the stomach can be made much smaller by inverting the stomach into itself, decreasing the space available for food inside. Various ways to do this were tried in studies on animals and patients. Mostly this involved pushing in and inverting either the lesser curvature or the greater curvature into the rest of the stomach. Since it was feared that stitches alone wouldn't hold the stomach in an inverted position, the stomachs were wrapped tightly with plastic (polypropylene) mesh. This turned out to be a tedious and difficult operation. Sometimes the wrapping was too tight which wasn't too good for the patient, and sometimes the stomach "escaped" from the wrap. Several variations of this technique were tried, but it hasn't really worked out.

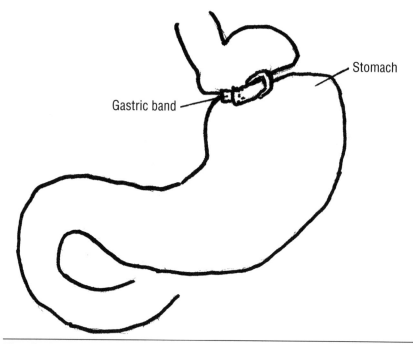

Gastric band

Stomach

Fig. 8. Gastric banding

Gastric banding is a different matter. The idea of tightening a plastic band around the stomach to create a small gastric pouch has its appeal, particularly since it is so nontraumatic. What I mean is that nothing penetrates the wall of the stomach, no stitches, no staples, no cutting. The basic idea is to put the band around the upper stomach and then tighten it as you would tighten a belt around your waist (Fig. 8). This provides a small stoma between the upper and lower parts of the stomach. How high the band is placed on the stomach determines how small the upper part will be, and how tight the band is secured will determine how narrow the stoma will be. The stomach assumes an hour-glass shape.

These operations were first performed in the early 1980s, and various plastic materials, such as nylon, Dacron, polypropylene mesh, and silastic have been used for the bands. These bands are made about 1 centimeter wide, and are usually tightened to create a stoma about 12 or 13 mm wide. Technically, these operations are simpler to perform than the stapling operations. But there are some complications that have occurred.

These have included obstruction of the stomach from the bands, enlargement of the pouch, and, most seriously, erosion of the band through the stomach wall to the inside. This is similar to the problems that surgeons have had when they have tried to reinforce the stomas of the gastroplasties and gastric bypasses, as we described above. The erosion complication is not all that common, but when it occurs it can be serious.

I had one patient who had had a banding operation referred to me because of one of these complications. She was complaining of abdominal pain and vomiting, and to make matters worse, she had gained back 60 of the 80 pounds that she had lost. When I operated on her, I found that the plastic band had eroded into the interior of the stomach, and that it had become wrapped tightly around an area of the stomach's lining. Even when I opened the stomach I could not remove the band. What a nightmare! I eventually had to cut out and remove part of the stomach. When our pathologists examined the part of the stomach that was removed they described severe congestion, inflammation, swelling, and areas of bleeding in the stomach lining. I finally managed to do a gastric bypass on the remaining part of the stomach. Recovery was slow, but she eventually did well.

I am not sure what the future holds for gastric banding. One doesn't hear too much about it these days in the professional literature, although I know that some surgeons still do this procedure and are enthusiastic. I remain skeptical, but I am willing to be convinced.

VERTICAL-BANDED GASTROPLASTY

There is one operation that makes use of a plastic band for limiting the size of the gastric-pouch outlet. This is the *vertical-banded gastroplasty*, first described by Mason in 1981 (Fig. 9). Mason continued to try more innovative approaches in an effort to come up with the perfect operation for morbid obesity. His vertical-banded gastroplasty has been widely accepted by surgeons, and may well be the most popular of all operations for obesity. I think its major appeal is that it is a relatively easy operation to perform, with very little dissection needed. In this operation, a round "window" is made completely through the stomach with a special instrument. The staples are then placed in a vertical fashion, from this window extending up to the upper part of the stomach just to the left of where the esophagus joins the stomach. So the stapling is vertical rather than hori-

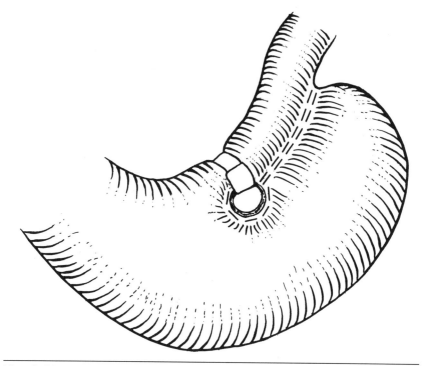

Fig. 9. Vertical-banded gastroplasty

zontal across the stomach. This vertical stapling results in a very small, narrow, up-and-down pouch, which has been measured by some as 19 cubic centimeters in capacity, slightly more than one tablespoon can hold. The resulting outlet or stoma is controlled in size by encircling it with a Marlex (polypropylene mesh) band.

While the vertical-banded gastroplasty is certainly a very acceptable operation, it is not my favorite. I am concerned that liquids and possibly soft foods might empty out of the stomach too rapidly because of the vertical nature of the pouch. With a horizontal pouch, I feel, the emptying of the stomach might be more delayed, and a longer-lasting feeling of fullness after eating would occur. I'm not sure whether this is true, but in several good studies by Pories et al.,[1] Sugarman et al.,[2] and Fobi and Fleming[3] that have been done comparing the effects of the vertical-banded gastroplasty with those of the gastric bypass, the latter operation has resulted in a greater loss of weight. Furthermore, although the vertical-banded operation is easier to perform, both operations have a very similar rate of complications such as gastric leaks, stomal stenosis, and wound infections. I feel that there is no advantage to the vertical-banded gastroplasty.

Some surgeons have tried to separate out two different types of patients: the high-calorie sweet eaters and the overeaters, and have said that one of these operations is best for one type of patient, and the other operation is best for the other. In my opinion, this distinction is artificial. I don't trust what many patients tell me about their eating habits, and many tell me that they overeat everything including sweets. So I stick with my loop gastric bypass, which has served me and my patients well for a long time—at least until a new procedure convinces me otherwise.

NOTES

1. E. J. Pories et al., "The Effectiveness of Gastric Bypass (GB) over Gastric Partitioning (GP) in Morbid Obesity (MO): Consequence of Distal Gastric and Duodenal Exclusion?" *Annals of Surgery* 186 (1982): 389–99.

2. H. T. Sugarman et al., "Weight Loss with Vertical Banded Gastroplasty and Roux-Y Gastric Bypass for Morbid Obesity with Selective versus Random Assignment," *American Journal of Surgery* 157 (1989): 93–100.

3. M. A. L. Fobi and A. W. Fleming, "Vertical Banded Gastroplasty vs Gastric Bypass in the Treatment of Obesity," *Journal of the National Medical Association* 78 (1986): 1091–98.

16

Gastric Bypass: My Syracuse Experience

Thought depends absolutely on the stomach, but in spite of that, those who have the best stomachs are not the best thinkers.

—Voltaire

The first gastric bypass I performed was in the spring of 1978 in Syracuse. I had been thinking about starting to do this operation earlier because of the good reports I had heard about others who had performed it, but most of my intestinal-bypass patients were doing so well that I was a little reluctant to make a change. I liked to think that my patients were doing well because I kept in close contact with them, and was able to treat all complications early before they became serious. But I did want to start doing some of these gastric bypasses so that I could make my own comparisons as to the worth of each operation.

During this time, in the late 1970s there was considerable controversy among surgeons as to which was better, the intestinal or the gastric bypass. Believe it or not, this often resulted in heated debates, sometimes becoming very emotional. Facts and truth were sometimes stretched to try to convince the surgical world that a particular operation was the best. I became very skeptical of the whole affair, and I wanted to make up my mind based on my own experience.

One of the things that finally pushed me into learning how to do the gastric bypass was an experience I had with one of my patients. This involved a young woman in her mid-twenties who was morbidly obese. Her preoperative laboratory tests were relatively normal with only slight

124

abnormalities of her liver-function tests, similar to what we often find in obese patients. At her operation, to my surprise, her liver appeared to be extremely damaged by cirrhosis. She later admitted to me that she had been an alcoholic since her teenage years. I removed a piece of liver as a biopsy, and sent it to the pathologist, asking for a frozen section, which allowed immediate microscopic examination of the specimen. The pathologist said it looked terrible. I had a conference in the operating room with the pathologist and a gastroenterologist who was very knowledgeable about liver disease. We all realized that the liver worsens during the first few months after an intestinal bypass, so we agreed that the bypass should not be done. When the patient awakened from the anesthesia, I explained the situation to her. It was then that she told me about her alcoholism.

I told her not to give up hope, that there was another operation, the gastric bypass, that apparently could be done safely on patients with liver disease. I checked this out with several surgeons who had experience with gastric bypasses. The patient returned home and soon after became pregnant. I planned to do her gastric bypass after she had her baby. But late in pregnancy she developed toxemia, a very serious complication of pregnancy. The decision was made to perform a Caesarean section. I was called into the operating room by the obstetricians to help with the operation on this extremely obese woman. She died a few days later as a result of the toxemia, the liver disease, and her obesity.

In the meantime, I had traveled to the University of Kansas Medical School where I scrubbed in on, and observed several gastric bypasses performed by surgeons who were friends of mine. I asked many questions and collected good information from them, not only about the actual technique of doing these operations, but also about the care of the patients after the procedure. I returned to Syracuse ready to start my gastric-bypass experience.

I continued to meet most of my patients in group sessions, with five or six patients in each group. But now I described both the intestinal and the gastric bypass to them, including the benefits and complications. The patients themselves decided whether or not to have an operation, and which of the two procedures to undergo. Since the most common side effect of the intestinal bypass was diarrhea, and of the gastric bypass vomiting, it sometimes came down to a personal choice between the lesser of two uncomfortable postoperative effects. Occasionally I decided which operation to perform. Obviously patients with liver disease would undergo gastric bypass.

Around the time I started doing the gastric bypasses, the intestinal bypass was receiving very bad press, both from other doctors as well as from newspapers and the media. It's incredible to me how deep this negative impression became and how long it has lasted. There are still doctors who say to me when I tell them that I perform gastric bypasses, "Why do you want to do this operation? Don't you know that the patient will have terrible diarrhea?" Even when I tell them that they are referring to the intestinal bypass, and that the gastric operation does not cause diarrhea, they look at me in disbelief.

After a few years of experience with the gastric bypass it became obvious to me that these patients made a much more rapid recovery from the operation than those who had an intestinal bypass. I did feel at first that the gastric-bypass patients did not lose as much weight as the others, but in time, with more results to analyze, I found that the results were very similar. The major difference was the lack of early and late complications from the gastric bypass. I could always tell which operation the patient had on the first postoperative visit to my office. The patients had to walk down a long corridor to get to my room. Some patients walked slowly, with great effort needed to reach my door. They were the intestinal-bypass patients. Other patients moved briskly, almost effortlessly, with a good healthy pace. They had had the gastric bypass, and had recovered most of their strength. The difference was striking.

From the first, I found the gastric bypass to be an interesting, but sometimes difficult operation. With the bypass, a liver biopsy, and an appendectomy, the operative time was almost five hours at first, but as my experience with this procedure improved, the operating time decreased to about two hours.

Both the gastric- and intestinal-bypass patients were housed on the same surgical floor. The nurses very quickly learned how to take care of this new group of patients. They could basically tell which patient had what operation by the presence of either diarrhea or vomiting after a few postoperative days.

GASTRIC-BYPASS PATIENTS

I continued to receive referrals from doctors all over central New York State and surrounding areas. I even began to get some referrals of patients from the doctors at my hospital, the Upstate Medical Center. From 1978 to 1982, I performed about 125 of these gastric-bypass operations. In most respects these patients were similar to those who had undergone the intestinal bypass. The age range was from fifteen to fifty-four years, with an average age of thirty-seven years. There were many more women, outnumbering the men seven to one. The range in weight was from 223 to 549 pounds, with an average of 308 pounds. Actually, there were some patients who weighed much less, as low as 126 pounds, but these were patients who were being converted from an intestinal to a gastric bypass, usually because of major complications.

The gastric-bypass patients had medical and physical problems relating to their obesity similar to those of the earlier intestinal-bypass patients. About a third had high blood pressure. Abnormal blood sugar levels were also common, apparent in more than a third of patients. Seven patients were diabetics requiring daily insulin injections, and several others were taking pills to control their diabetes. At least 40 percent of the patients complained of chronic back pain or arthritis of their hips, knees, or ankles. Nearly one-third of patients had elevated levels of blood cholesterol or triglycerides. Finally, gallbladder disease was very common, in almost 40 percent, with about half of them needing removal of the gallbladder at the time of the gastric bypass. The other half already had their gallbladders removed before coming to see me. These figures are almost identical to those of the intestinal-bypass patients.

POSTOPERATIVE MANAGEMENT

After the gastric bypass, patients were not permitted to eat or drink for about four or five days. Intravenous fluids were given during this time, and the nasogastric tube extending from outside of the nose down to the stomach was kept on suction to remove any air or fluid in the stomach. On the fourth or fifth postoperative day, an X-ray of the stomach was performed. This involved swallowing a rather unpleasant but safe radiopaque dye called *gastrografin*. If the X-ray showed no abnormalities, the nasogastric tube was removed and the patient was started on small amounts of a liquid diet. Most patients tolerated this well and were ready to leave the hospital by the sixth or seventh postoperative day.

After about three weeks on liquids the patients were started on a regular diet. At first the patients were very limited as to what and how much they could eat. Gradually they were able to tolerate a greater variety of foods and the amount also gradually increased. When I say a small amount of food, I really mean it. Patients would tell me that they could only eat two or three mouthfuls of food without feeling uncomfortably stuffed. If they ate one additional bite of food, it was too much, and vomiting would usually follow. Or if they didn't vomit, they would be extremely uncomfortable for hours.

Under these circumstances, as you can imagine, they certainly lost weight. Weight loss was fastest at first, usually 8 to 12 percent during the first month, and then very gradually slower as the weeks and months went by. Their weight usually leveled off at about one year after the operation. Why did these patients lose weight? The obvious and correct answer relates to their caloric intake. We did a careful study on dietary intake before and after surgery. (I talked about this in chapter 12 on intestinal bypass.) This group of gastric-bypass patients averaged 6,000 calories per day *before* surgery: including 699 grams of carbohydrates, 206 grams of protein, and 251 grams of fat. We unfortunately didn't measure their caloric intake during their month on liquids, but it was undoubtedly very low. At three months after surgery, the caloric intake averaged only 740 calories per day, with 73 grams of carbohydrate, 35 grams of protein, and 36 grams of fat. Quite a difference! At six months after surgery, their caloric intake had risen to about 1,200 calories. We estimated that they probably leveled off at 1,300 to 1,500 calories per day by one year, which is a good maintenance figure for these patients.

WEIGHT LOSS

The average weight loss for these patients was about 32 percent of their starting weight. While this looks to be a little less than that occurring after the intestinal bypass, it is statistically about the same. Some patients lost more, up to about 55 percent of starting weight. We did have some failures, and relative failures, but let me first talk about some of the successes.

PATIENTS' STORIES

I always like to think about one of my patients, Georgia, who had a very attractive manner about her even though she weighed almost 250 pounds. She was in her thirties and was about 5 feet 6 inches tall. Before her operation she hung up a large poster of the actress Natalie Wood in a bathing suit on the wall opposite her bed in the hospital room. This was meant to inspire her. She said to me, "This is how I will look a year from now." I didn't want to discourage her, but that would have meant a spectacular weight loss, and it just doesn't happen that often after the surgery. I told her that she probably would lose a lot of weight, but not to be discouraged if she didn't quite get to Natalie Wood's size. When I saw her last, about two years after her operation, she weighed 122 pounds and looked just about as great as she had hoped. Obviously a success.

Another memorable patient was Donald, a forty-year-old man who was 5 feet 11 inches tall and weighed almost 300 pounds. He was suffering from one of the most interesting complications of morbid obesity, the Pickwickian syndrome. He underwent a gastric bypass, and his operation was very difficult. As a complication of his operation an abscess developed deep in his abdominal cavity and he had to be reoperated on to drain it. Now the interesting thing to me was his profession—a lawyer. Doctors sometimes get very nervous treating lawyers, and I was a little worried myself. It took a long time for his infection to heal completely, although he was able to be discharged from the hospital after a relatively short time. In spite of the infection he did well. His weight eventually dropped down to 173 pounds (a 41 percent weight loss) and his Pickwickian syndrome completely disappeared.

Another patient, Florence, had been referred to me by one of our neurologists. Her weight was about 255 pounds and she had elevated levels of blood cholesterol and triglycerides. He sent her to me because she suffered from blurred vision and headaches. The neurologist had diagnosed a condition called *pseudotumor cerebri* which can be caused by extreme obesity, although there are other causes as well. A gastric bypass was performed and her weight went down to 182 pounds (a 29 percent loss). The symptoms disappeared, but every so often she again complained of headaches, dizziness, and pain in her eyes. All of her neurological exams were normal, as compared to her preoperative exams. She was probably cured of her pseudotumor cerebri, but the occasional return of symptoms was upsetting, at least to me.

There were several very heavy men, weighing well over 400 pounds, who had very good results from their gastric bypasses. This was similar to the good results I had with the intestinal bypass on some of these superobese men. Gordon, a dairy farmer, weighed 497 pounds and suffered from high blood pressure, breathing problems, and arthritis, especially involving his knees. When I saw him last, over a year after his surgery, his weight had dropped to 232 pounds, which was an excellent 53 percent loss. Another man, Bernard, who also had problems with his knees weighed 440 pounds before his operation. His weight went down to 236 pounds (a very substantial 46 percent loss). And a third man I operated on, Simon, weighed 416 pounds, suffering from the Pickwickian syndrome and back and knee pains. He was a manager of a local supermarket and was having increasing problems with his work and his daily life. His gastric bypass was successful, with his weight decreasing to 267 pounds (a 39 percent weight loss). More importantly, his breathing difficulties disappeared, as did the back and knee pain. These were all great results. I also had some failures, and there were certainly patients who experienced some complications, as you will see in chapter 17.*

CONVERSION OPERATIONS

I do want to mention another special group of patients that I operated on. These were people who had what I call the "conversion operation." They underwent a conversion from the intestinal bypass to the gastric bypass, and this was done for a variety of reasons relating to problems from the intestinal bypass. I finally got the feeling that possibly 50 percent of patients with intestinal bypasses would have to undergo conversion to gastric bypass because of these problems, another 25 percent had intestinal-bypass problems but were coping with them without need for reoperation, and 25 percent were doing well without complications. These percentages reflect my own personal estimates.

At any rate, many patients have needed these conversion operations. After several procedures, we learned that, if possible, the reversal of the intestinal bypass and the creation of the gastric bypass should be done at the same time, as one operation. This meant that if the patient was suffering from one of the more serious complications it should be treated aggressively to get the patient in the best possible shape for the operation. For example, if liver disease had developed, the patient needed good nutritional support, frequently given intravenously, to improve the functioning of the liver before undergoing reoperation.

---

*I'm going to put off discussing this until the next chapter, my New York experience, where I'll lump together all the good and bad of my gastric-bypass experiences. As you'll see, there was much more good than bad, and we all learned how to handle most of the problems, and actually how to decrease their occurrence.

The intestinal-bypass reversal and creation of the gastric bypass should be done as a single operation because of its relationship to the patient's regaining of weight. Patients began to regain weight as soon as the intestine was restored to its original state. An example was Gwen, a thirty-five-year-old woman who had an intestinal bypass done in a nearby hospital when she weighed 285 pounds. Her weight loss was excessive, and when she reached 114 pounds the same surgeons reversed the bypass. She then started to regain weight very rapidly, nearly six pounds per week. When she came to see me, she weighed 180 pounds. I performed a gastric bypass, and ultimately her weight stabilized at about 150 pounds, which was an acceptable weight for her.

Sometimes this conversion operation was done for the wrong reason or for no reason at all. There was, and still is some irrational hysteria about intestinal bypasses. Some doctors think that every patient should have it undone, even if they are doing well. I don't agree. I had one patient, a thirty-four-year-old woman whose weight decreased from 414 pounds to 171 pounds. She had many problems from the operation at first, but seemed to be coping with them. I heard from her a few years after I left Syracuse. She had been convinced to undergo reoperation to get rid of the intestinal bypass, and someone did a gastroplasty operation which did not work very well. The pouch and the stoma both stretched, and she started to regain weight at a rapid pace. I felt this was a shame since the conversion operation was probably unnecessary. I reoperated on her when her weight had climbed to 236 pounds, converting her gastroplasty to a gastric bypass. The recovery period was difficult and she didn't have an easy time, but when I last heard from her she reported that her weight was back down to 171 pounds and she was doing well and enjoying her thin life.

Most patients who underwent the conversion operation had it done because of multiple intestinal-bypass complications. One patient was a forty-three-year-old man, Arthur, who weighed 338 pounds. He had diabetes requiring daily insulin injections, high blood pressure, and heart disease. I did an intestinal bypass, and immediately his diabetes improved without the need for insulin. But about three months later he began to suffer from kidney stones related to the intestinal bypass. The diarrhea was a problem, but his worst discomfort was due to bloating from a tremendous amount of intestinal gas. I had never seen this to so great an extent. Nothing seemed to work to control these problems. I reoperated on him nine months after his original operation, converting him to a gastric bypass. His weight had dropped down to 228 pounds, and a year after his conversion operation his weight had reached 177 pounds. This was a very good 48 percent loss. Even more important, his diabetes and high blood pressure were both gone, as was the problem of excessive gas.

Another patient, Alice, who underwent the conversion operation originally weighed 481 pounds. She was a thirty-two-year-old woman who also had high blood pressure, and her laboratory tests suggested the beginning of diabetes. She had many problems after her intestinal bypass, but eventually she improved, and her weight decreased to 178 pounds. About six years after the operation she began to develop a major calcium deficiency in her blood. We tried huge doses of calcium supplements, vitamin D, and other medications, but nothing worked. Periodically she would come into the Emergency Room with severe muscle spasms (tetany), particularly of her hands. This would respond to intravenously administered calcium. Between the tetany and an increase in diarrhea, we felt the time had come for a conversion to a gastric bypass. After surgery the calcium and diarrhea vanished. She regained some weight, but leveled off in the low 200s.

The conversion operation was done on another patient, Helen, who was suffering from vomiting, diarrhea, chronic fatigue, and easy bruising of her skin about a year and a half after undergoing the intestinal bypass. Individually these problems were not serious, but together they constituted a situation where she was just not feeling very well. The weight of this forty-six-year-old woman had dropped 49 percent to 142 pounds. She recovered very nicely after the conversion to gastric bypass although her weight rose slightly to 167 pounds. This was still a very acceptable 41 percent loss. And of greater importance, all her symptoms disappeared.

One patient had a more unusual situation. Paul was thirty-one years old and weighed 461 pounds before his intestinal-bypass surgery. Everything went well after surgery for about three years. Then he began to develop dizziness, blurred vision, and incoordination. The neurologists felt he had an unusual condition called d-lactic acidosis and conversion to a gastric bypass was suggested. The conversion was completed and soon the symptoms disappeared. His weight leveled off to 217 pounds, a 52 percent weight loss.

A more common reason for the conversion operation was related to the development of "bypass arthritis." This occurred in a patient who was thirty-five years old and weighed 280 pounds before her intestinal bypass. About six years after the operation she developed arthralgias that involved several joints, but moved around from joint to joint. This began to cause her considerable pain and trouble, and she was treated with a variety of drugs. Eventually she was placed on adrenal steroids (anti-inflammatory agents). We knew that reversal of the intestinal bypass would totally eliminate this problem. The conversion operation was performed with the expected success.

The most recent conversion operation I have done was seventeen years after the original intestinal bypass. As you can see, serious complications resulting from the intestinal bypass can occur long after the operation. This patient, Harvey, developed increased diarrhea, potassium deficiency, weakness, and possible early liver disease, in spite of a fairly benign course for the first fifteen years. The conversion operation appears to have eliminated all of these problems.

Sometimes the conversion operation does not produce the desired result. I wrote in chapter 13 about Lily, who developed arthritis after her intestinal bypass. The arthritis specialists who examined her were not sure whether this was bypass arthritis or a newly developed rheumatoid arthritis. After she had the conversion operation, the arthritis remained, and the obvious conclusion focused on rheumatoid arthritis.

One of my patients had the usual problems after the intestinal bypass, but experienced similar problems after the gastric bypass. She was Audrey, who was forty-five years old and weighed 275 pounds. She had high blood pressure, heart disease, and diabetes, which was treated by antidiabetic pills. Her major problem after the intestinal bypass was vomiting. All her X-rays were normal, and we never could find the reason for her vomiting. She did have serious emotional problems which possibly could have caused the vomiting, but we were never sure. Her weight dropped down to 147 pounds, but the vomiting persisted. A year after the first operation, a conversion operation was done. She again experienced problems with vomiting, which is common after a gastric bypass, but since her weight dropped further to 119 pounds, readmission to the hospital with nutritional support was necessary. She finally improved, and gained some weight. Then she gained more weight, which made us suspect a different problem. An X-ray of her stomach revealed that the staples had pulled apart. We had to operate again to restaple her stomach. She continued to vomit but, mercifully, it stopped. The last time I saw her she weighed 145 pounds and was improved. It is an understatement to say that she had a difficult time.

Yet another patient of mine developed a very interesting problem after her conversion operation. She was fifty years old when she had the intestinal bypass, and she weighed 356 pounds. Most of her preoperative problems involved arthritis. Five years after the operation we performed a conversion. This was decided upon because she suffered from kidney stones, increased diarrhea, and bloating. Also her weight, which had decreased to 186 pounds, had started to rise, and reached 227 pounds. Her orthopedist felt that she could be a candidate for a much-needed orthopedic operation to help her arthritis if she could only lose more weight. The conversion operation went well and her weight did drop somewhat, to 208 pounds. The problem was that she developed severe constipation. This was very unusual.

Remember, after the intestinal bypass she had only about 10 percent of her small intestine functioning, the rest was being bypassed. When the intestine was put back together again in the conversion operation, she had 100 percent of the intestine functioning. It appeared that her intestine was then functioning too well, absorbing too much of the liquid in her stool thus causing a severe, hard constipation. With a great deal of effort, we came up with the right medication for her, and the problem relented.

I did have a patient, Ashley, somewhat later, in my New York practice, who also developed severe constipation after a conversion operation. Her condition was even more difficult to treat. No medication seemed to help. I finally read several articles in surgical journals that reported the use of a near-total removal of the large intestine as a treatment for severe, unrelenting constipation. I then performed this procedure on the patient, and much to my surprise it worked. Fortunately, serious constipation after conversion operations is rare. But why does it happen at all, and why is it not more common?

Another major reason for performing the conversion operation is to bring about additional weight loss. Some patients just did not lose enough weight from the intestinal bypass. The gastric bypass sometimes did a better job. One of my patients, Brittany, was a thirty-seven-year-old woman who weighed 253 pounds. After her intestinal bypass, the woman's weight leveled off much too early to 222 pounds. The 31-pound weight loss was only 12 percent, much less than we normally achieve. To make things worse, she started to regain some of this lost weight, and within three and a half years after the first operation her weight was back up to 242 pounds. The conversion operation was performed in the hope of improving her results. The last time I saw her, four months later, her weight was down to 192 pounds. She missed her next appointments, but she wrote me a year later that she weighed between 138 and 145 pounds and felt exceptionally good.

Another success story involved a thirty-three-year-old hospital nurse who weighed 238 pounds before surgery. After the intestinal bypass her weight leveled off at 190 pounds, only a 20 percent loss. A year later, I reoperated on her, shortening her intestinal bypass even more. With this her weight dropped only to 178 pounds while her diarrhea became excessive. A year after the second operation I again operated on her, performing a conversion to a gastric bypass. This appeared to work better, and seven months later her weight had decreased to 148 pounds, a 39 percent loss from her original weight. It actually worked too well. She got married, moved to California, and our hospital lost a good nurse.

Unfortunately, sometimes the conversion operation does not result in additional weight loss. I performed an intestinal bypass on a thirty-six-year-old diabetic woman, Leslie, who weighed 326 pounds. Twenty months after the surgery she weighed 214 pounds, a good 34 percent weight loss. But then she started to regain some of the weight, and at a point forty-four months later, the weight had risen to 252 pounds. It was decided to proceed with a conversion operation. Four months after the surgery she weighed 232 pounds, but started to gain weight again. Her weight rose to 291 pounds and then dropped back to 279 pounds. Nothing seemed to work for her to maintain a long-term weight objective. I have heard other surgeons say that some patients just don't achieve a stable weight range regardless of what operation is done.

The final patient I'll discuss had just the reverse problem, too much weight loss after the intestinal bypass, and little change after her conversion surgery. Joan was thirty-nine years old and weighed 269 pounds. After the intestinal bypass she had considerable problems with vomiting and then diarrhea. She also had severe emotional problems. Her weight went down rapidly, and at fifteen months after surgery she weighed 127 pounds. Because of all her problems, including the very excessive weight loss, a conversion operation was performed. With the expected postoperative vomiting, her weight went down further, reaching a low point of 106 pounds at three and a half months. She then started to improve, and her weight started to go up. But a few weeks later she was involved in an automobile accident, after which she experienced nausea, headaches, and dizziness. The neurologists gave a diagnosis of postconcussive syndrome. When I last saw her two and a half years after the original operation her weight had risen only to 133 pounds, a 51 percent loss.

As time goes by, I seem to be doing fewer and fewer conversion operations. Have all the intestinal-bypass patients been reoperated on? Or have we finally reached a point where all of those patients who are slated for the development of serious problems have already had them, and the rest of the intestinal-bypass patients are doing well and will continue to do so? I hope the latter is so, but I wouldn't bet on it.

The addition of gastric bypass to the arsenal of the antiobese surgeon was a radical one. I had to learn a new operative technique and learn how to manage these patients. As you will see in the next chapter, I started to do the gastric bypass exclusively since it appeared to be a safe technique as well as an effective one.

17

Gastric Bypass: My New York Experience

Serenely full, the epicure would say,
Fate cannot harm me,—I have dined today.
—Sydney Smith, "Lady Holland's Memoir"

At the end of 1982, I moved to New York City. My children were all grown up, and my wife and I decided that we would like to move back to New York where we both were born and raised. I accepted the position of chief of surgery at one of the city hospitals and professor of surgery at New York Medical College. I also joined the staff of the Westchester County Medical Center. The Westchester County Medical Center is located in Valhalla, New York, on a nice grassy plot of land. The hospital is relatively new and attractive. Its nursing care is particularly good, and it's usually a very pleasant place to work.

When I left Syracuse, business had been "booming." I had a list of about sixty to seventy patients who were waiting for appointments for the gastric-bypass surgery. The word had finally gotten around that this was a safe, effective operation, and I was receiving referrals from patients and doctors outside of Syracuse, and also, believe it or not, from some of the doctors in my own hospital. When I moved to New York, I realized that I would have to start all over again attracting patients and physicians interested in this type of surgery. The chief of surgery at the hospital had done this type of operation on a few patients, but he was not really interested in specializing. He assured me that he would send all prospective patients to me, including any of his patients who needed conversions.

The first patient I operated on, in January 1983, was one of his former patients, Fred, who needed a conversion. The young man had weighed more than 600 pounds when he underwent the first surgery. He was a graduate student at one of the universities, but because of his excessive weight he was unable to continue his studies. At one point, while he was in the hospital awaiting surgery, he apparently changed his mind, and left the building. Some of his doctors and nurses ran after him, chasing him around the block, and finally convincing him to return. I don't know how difficult the first operation was, but I do know that they strapped two operating tables together to accommodate his bulk. The operation, a gastroplasty, was successful and his weight dropped down to 380 pounds. But gradually his weight started to climb, and it appeared that the outlet stoma had dilated. He was referred to me for further surgery. At the time he weighed 402 pounds. During the second operation I converted his gastroplasty to a gastric bypass. This proved successful. About a year after the reoperation, he weighed 231 pounds. He was back in school, and was also driving a taxi after school to make some money. That's the last I saw of him, but I did receive some news about him from one of our surgery residents. This former patient of ours had completed his schooling, and was now on the teaching staff of the university. When asked about the teacher's appearance, the resident said that the teacher was a little heavy, but that you "wouldn't look at him twice" because of his weight.

OPERATIVE MANAGEMENT

The operations I performed in New York were the same gastric bypasses I had done in Syracuse (Fig. 10), but over the years a number of technical modifications had been made. Actually, the operation continued to change, but only in minor ways that we surgeons hoped made it safer and more effective.

Without becoming too technical, there are some aspects of the operation that I should describe. First, I never used two operating tables, even to accommodate my biggest patients. It put me too far away from the patient. Instead, I used the arm boards to provide some extra space for the patient. The arm boards are usually placed at right angles from the table so that the patient can place his or her arms in a comfortable position. When the arm boards were placed alongside the table, and not at right angles, they added about five or six inches of room on each side.

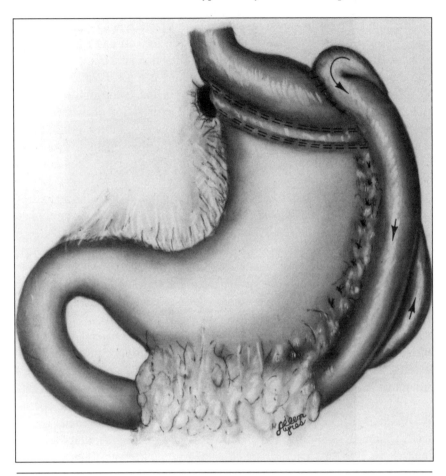

Fig. 10. Gastric bypass (as I do it). (Reproduced by permission from *General Surgery* 2, revised edition, edited by John J. Byrne, M.D., and Harry S. Goldsmith, M.D. [Philadelphia: Harper & Row, 1984])

After the patient was anesthetized, a five-to-six-inch incision was made starting at the end of the ribs in the midline, going down toward the navel. Only the skin itself was cut by the scalpel. The very deep fatty layer beneath the skin, which can measure several inches in depth, was not cut. Instead, it was pulled apart by me and my resident assistant on the opposite side of the table. While this may sound painful if not grotesque, it actually isn't. It is fast, usually bloodless because blood vessels don't cross the midline, and it took us down to the *linea alba* which is the thick fibrous midportion between the abdominal muscles on the left and right sides. If you cut all the way through with a scalpel, the linea alba could be hard to find through all the fat, so the pulling technique is a good one.

The incision into the abdominal cavity is made through this linea alba, avoiding the abdominal muscles. A full exploration of the abdomen is then made. As mentioned earlier, I usually do a liver biopsy (since there is almost always some inflammation and fat that has infiltrated into the liver) and an appendectomy if the appendix can be safely reached through this incision. Remember, our incision is fairly high in the abdomen and sometimes the appendix is very low on the right side. It could be particularly hard to get to the appendix in some very tall men. It is certainly not an absolute necessity to remove the appendix in these patients.

The actual performance of the gastric bypass can be difficult at times. Some of these difficulties are related to the depth of the abdomen measured from the front to the back. If it is very deep, the operation can be harder.

During the operation, all of the blood vessels and supportive tissues of the upper part of the left side of the stomach are tied and cut. This is the hard part of the operation since these vessels and tissues extend deep down in the abdominal cavity almost underneath the ribs. Once the tissues and vessels are separated and cut, we are able to reach the esophagus just coming out of the chest cavity into the abdomen. We are then able to pull the rounded, bulbous part of the left side of the stomach down into the operative field so that connecting it to the jejunum can be safely done under direct vision. In doing this, the upper part of the stomach assumes a triangular shape. The surgical residents named this "Ackerman's triangle."

In doing this part of the operation, one has to be particularly careful not to injure the spleen. In the experience of most surgeons who have done gastric bypasses splenic injuries have occurred, and in as many as 5 to 6 percent of patients in some series the spleen had to be removed because of injury and uncontrolled splenic bleeding. In my early experience I had several cases where injuries to the spleen occurred. I was able to stop the bleeding with the help of agents like thrombin, which promote blood clotting, placed right on the injured area. Only once have I had to remove a spleen in one of these operations. For a long time I did not understand why these injuries occurred. In none of my operations where an injury of the spleen occurred was I anywhere near the spleen at the time of injury. How could it have happened? It finally dawned on me that organs are connected in the abdomen by fibrous bands and ligaments.

When the stomach was pulled or retracted to afford exposure during the operation, fibrous, fatty tissue connecting the stomach and spleen was also being pulled. The covering or capsule of the spleen could get torn, and major bleeding could result. Once I realized this, and lightened up on the retraction of the stomach, the incidence of splenic injuries decreased.

After the stomach dissection was completed and the upper part of the stomach could be gently pulled downward, the connection was made between it and the jejunum. The upper part of the jejunum was identified and was gently pulled upward so that the two organs lay side by side. We had a sterile ruler on the operating table that allowed us to measure 8 millimeters for the openings in the stomach and intestine. These organs were then meticulously sewn together to provide a very small, 8 mm connection. Then the stapling instrument was placed across the stomach, from below the gastrointestinal connection on the left side to the gastroesophageal junction on the right side, in a slanted fashion, leaving more left-sided stomach in the resulting pouch.

The stapler I originally used fired thirty-three small, stainless-steel staples across the stomach, in two close-together rows. As we learned after a while, these two rows were not enough, because sometimes the staples pulled apart, permitting food to fill the entire stomach. So we started using the stapler twice, giving us four rows with sixty-six staples. This wasn't much better, so we added a row of stitches placed just beyond the staples. We still had occasional problems. Happily, the company that made these stapling instruments came up with the obvious, but ultimate instrument, the TA-90B, which fires sixty-six staples from one cartridge, giving four close together, parallel rows. I am not sure why this worked out better than what we used before, but it has. I have used this stapler since March 1987 without difficulty.

These instruments are now well made and are quite sophisticated in construction. It wasn't so in the early years. I remember in the late 1970s that the instruments had many pieces that had to be put together accurately so that the stapler could function. Sometimes these pieces would fall off, and sometimes the whole instrument would seem to fall apart. In some operations I found myself catching these pieces just before they fell on the floor. It was like a slapstick comedy, everyone grabbing here and there to prevent contamination of the various parts. And in these early years in Syracuse only one operating-room nurse knew how to put the staple instrument back together. One day she was at lunch when our instrument fell apart. I remember everyone screaming, "Get Chris, get Chris!" Fortunately, things are better now.

While most of these gastric-bypass operations are rather straightforward, some can be fairly difficult. Strangely enough, there is no direct relationship just between weight and degree of difficulty. Some of the operations on the heaviest patients, those in the 400- to 500-pound category, are reasonably easy, while some on 200-pound patients are very difficult. Depth of the abdomen, as noted above, is one factor, but it is often unpredictable as to how difficult the operation might be. I started rating the degree of difficulty of the operation on a scale of from 1 to 10 just to see if there is any relationship between difficulty and complications. There isn't. The easiest cases are rated as 1, and they are a delight. The hardest one rated 8 or 9, and the less I remember about them the better, although even these patients do well.

All patients have a long tube placed (the nasogastric tube) in their nose and threaded down the esophagus to the stomach. This is always put in by the anesthesiologists when the patients are asleep during the operation. The tube is put on suction to empty out the stomach of any gas or fluid. At first I used the standard plastic tubes that are used in most abdominal surgical cases. But then I learned about perforations occurring in the stomach that were believed to be caused by pressure from the hard tips of these tubes. These were called "pistol shot" perforations, because they were small and round like a bullet hole. I immediately turned to the old-fashioned red rubber tubes which are not as efficient in some ways, but at least they haven't caused any perforations.

As I gradually became more familiar with the operation, the time in surgery shortened. The upper left side of the stomach, going all the way up to where the stomach and esophagus meet, was often a difficult area to expose, even sometimes in less obese patients. This is really underneath the lower ribs, and a surgeon can't pull the ribs back to gain better expose. Also, in some patients the rib cage is long and close together on both sides, leaving a relatively small area in which to make an incision and operate. All of this, coupled with the depth factor mentioned above plus the tremendous amount of fat in the area, can make the operation difficult. From a surgical standpoint, the problem with the fat is that it simply gets in the way and has to be gently pushed aside to be able to perform the operation. Also, it tends to obscure everything, including the small arteries and veins going to the stomach and the spleen. These blood vessels are easily seen in thinner patients and they can be tied off if necessary to prevent any bleeding. In morbidly obese patients, I tie off some of these fatty areas where I know some blood vessels are present, but I couldn't always directly see the vessels.

As I mentioned above, we always "explore" or examine fully the abdominal cavity before proceeding with the operation. The reason for this, I think, is obvious. Sometimes we found things of considerable importance that have to be attended to. Cancer, for example. Some of these abnormalities are so small or early in their development that they can not be detected by physical exam or the usual tests. Even some of the larger problems were difficult to detect on physical exams because of the massive size of the patients. So this exploration is often very beneficial to the patient. In one patient, Ellen, we discovered a malignant lymphoma of the intestines. We removed this, and then performed the gastric bypass. The patient has done well from both parts of the operation. Another patient, Amber, had a cancer of the ovary that we found during a reoperation. This was a very early cancer, and she, too, has done well after it was removed. I have also had three patients who had benign ovarian teratomas found while we explored the lower abdomen. Two were the size of softballs, and one was smaller. Teratomas are interesting tumors that contain weird things such as hair and teeth. They can be malignant or benign. Fortunately all three of these tumors were benign. One other patient had a rare type of benign adrenal tumor. The more common things we find include hernias around the navel, ovarian cysts, and gallbladder stones.

When we close the abdomen at the end of the operation, a soft rubber drain is put in and around the stapled area, and brought to the outside through a small opening made in the abdominal wall just to the left of the incision. The purpose of this drain is to let us know if there is any leakage of fluid from the stomach or intestine that might cause peritonitis. The drain also provides a passageway which permits any of these fluids to flow to the outside of the body rather than just staying inside the abdominal cavity where an abscess might develop.

We close the abdominal wall with stitches made of Vicryl, an artificial suture material that dissolves very slowly in the body. It is strong, easy to work with, and is well tolerated by the body. Then I insert two plastic drains in the fatty layer beneath the skin and these drains are brought to the outside through small openings made just below the incision. These drains are placed on suction to remove any fluid (serum) that develops in this space beneath the skin. The skin is closed with metallic clips rather than stitches.

Patients always wonder about the metal staples and all the other metallic clips we put in their bodies. "Will I be able to pass through the metal detectors in the airport?" The answer is yes. All of these staples and clips are very, very small. The stomach staples are so small that they are often difficult to see on X-rays.

POSTOPERATIVE MANAGEMENT

These operations, even the more difficult ones, generally go well. When the patients leave the operating room they are taken to the recovery room where they gradually wake up. They are pretty groggy for the next few hours, and much of this time is a blur to them. The nurses in recovery are very skillful and very sophisticated in managing the complicated monitoring equipment. This equipment allows continuous monitoring of all parts of the body, including the heart function, blood pressure, distribution of oxygen in the body, breathing functions, kidney function, and so on. Fortunately, these patients don't need the ultrasophisticated care given in the Intensive Care Units of the hospital. But I do like to keep my patients in recovery overnight whenever possible because there are more nurses per patient than on the regular hospital floors.

By the day after the operation patients go back to their regular hospital rooms but nourishment for the first few days is given intravenously. After a few days, when stomach and intestinal function begin to recover, I order an X-ray of the stomach—an upper GI (gastrointestinal) series for which the patient swallowed a dye called *gastrografin*. The X-ray gives three bits of information. First, it shows the size of the gastric pouch that we just made. Second, it reassures us that the stoma—the 8-mm connection that we made between the stomach and jejunum—is not blocked off by anything, and is functioning well. Third and most important, it shows that healing has occurred and no perforations or leakages are present. We then remove the patient's nasogastric tube, much to the patient's relief!

I then start the patients on a liquid diet. On the first day they are given one ounce of liquids, three times during the day. If this is tolerated, and it always seems to be, they move up to three ounces, three times a day. Now three ounces is not very much, but it does seem to be the capacity of their stomachs at this time. In fact, they can't just drink it all down in one gulp. They sip it slowly, sometimes taking as much as fifteen or twenty minutes to finish it off. At this point, it is now six or seven days after the operation, and most patients are ready to go home, unless there is a complication to attend to. Fortunately, complications of gastric bypass (unlike intestinal bypass) are very uncommon, so most patients go home.

Patients are sent home on a diet of three ounces of liquids, three times a day. The liquids include juices of any type, clear broths (not creamed soups), soda, tea, or coffee without cream (but they can use nondairy creamers), Jell-O, and ices (not ice cream). They are not allowed to drink milk or milk products since some patients have trouble tolerating them during this early period after the operation. Patients taking vitamins are advised to use the chewable variety. Most vitamin capsules or liquids have a terrible taste and smell, and may cause the gastric-bypass patients to increase their feeling of nausea, and even start vomiting.

After three weeks at home, patients come back to see me in my office. For the first two weeks they are usually very weak and tired, and really wonder if they did the right thing having this operation. But by the third week they begin to feel much better, and are usually glad to see me (I hope). At this time I take out their skin clips around the skin incision. For three weeks most patients worry about how painful it will be to have the skin clips removed, in spite of my reassurance that it wouldn't hurt. And it doesn't. There is a little gadget that makes the clips just pop right out without causing any real pain. I used to remove these clips after only one week, but I found that the skin on very obese patients sometimes begins to separate when the clips are removed so early. I would get frantic calls that the skin was starting to burst apart. It isn't really, but a little bit of separation can be very alarming to patients. With the clips in place for about a month, healing is excellent, and they aren't an inconvenience.

The other thing I do at this first postoperative visit is to switch them over to a regular diet. Now every surgeon seems to have his or her own ideas about dietary management for the gastric-bypass patient. Some put patients on regular food early, some prescribe liquids for longer periods, and some surgeons put patients on pureed foods or even baby foods. While the thought of patients eating baby foods doesn't appeal to me (or to them for that matter!), each surgeon develops what he or she considers to be the best postoperative diet.

I suggest to patients that they start on soft, bland foods. The two foods that most patients tolerate are mashed potatoes (without butter, sour cream, or anything) and crackers (e.g., saltines). Other suggested foods are cottage cheese, tuna fish (packed in water, not oil), cereals, puddings, egg salad (without mayonnaise), and apple sauce. Once they are tolerating most of these foods, I tell them to try other foods such as vegetables, fruits, cheese, chicken, fish, salads (no oily dressings), and low-fat milk. Patients are told that the final group of foods, those most difficult to tolerate, should not be tried until they are eating almost everything else. These foods include beef in any form; fried, greasy, spicy foods; and white bread and rice. Why white bread and rice? The answer is that while most foods chewed well break into small pieces that can pass through the narrow stoma that we create, some gummy foods such as white bread and rice just stick together in a clump and don't pass through this stoma. They just stay in the stomach and eventually get vomited out. So they're on the list of foods to avoid in the early stages.

The types of foods some patients start with can be really strange. It is difficult for me to understand why, psychologically, patients choose some of these foods. One patient claimed she could only tolerate peanut butter and liverwurst for the first few months. Another patient started with chili and tolerated it. I mentioned this to another patient as an example of what not to try, and she of course tried it and became very ill. Many patients are able to eat and tolerate pizza. Some patients tolerate pasta, at least the thick noodle types, but often not spaghetti and the thinner pasta types. Patients frequently say that they can eat a particular food on one day, but can't tolerate the same food a few days later. I even had one patient who claimed to drink the milk from one supermarket, but couldn't hold down the same brand of milk purchased from a different supermarket.

There does seem to be an emotional component to this toleration of food after the gastric bypass. Some patients, especially mothers of small or teenage children, say that if they eat with the rest of the family they frequently have trouble holding the food down, particularly if there is a lot of tension and stress during the meals. I tell these patients that they might have to eat separately from their families during the early period after surgery. I tell them, "Feed your family first, then get them out of the room, close the door, put the radio on, relax, and then eat." It seems to help. This is only necessary during the first days or weeks.

I give patients specific instructions how to eat. They are told to eat slowly, and chew everything well to a mushy consistency. After only two or three or four mouthfuls of food, they feel full. At that point they have to stop, even if they have a forkful of food ready to be eaten. When they feel full, there is absolutely no room left in their stomachs, and if they did take another bite of food they will not be able to hold it down. I tell my female patients that they will be cheap dates for a while, and will usually be able to eat off their husband's or boyfriend's plate in a restaurant. One surgeon I know gives his patients a card requesting the right to order children's portions in restaurants.

Gradually, gastric-bypass patients are able to increase the varieties of food they can eat, and also the amount of food. By the time weight loss slows down, they are usually able to eat virtually everything, and the amount increases to what I call a "plateful of food." This means some meat or fish and some vegetables, but not a second or third portion; or a sandwich, but not two or more; or most of a hamburger, not two or three or four. The patient's appetite, which is usually nonexistent at first, gradually comes back. Many regain their enjoyment of food, look forward to a nice meal, and seem to be satisfied because they are eating real food, not just picking, and they are eating what they *should* eat. Patient satisfaction is high.

Some patients experience changes in what they like to eat. One patient, Louise, who described herself as "a meat and potatoes person" before surgery, told me that she particularly looked forward to her nice salads. She hated salads before her operation. Some patients develop a strong dislike for sweets and desserts. One woman, Charlotte, told me that she had bought a pack of rolled candy and it had lasted a long time. Before her surgery she would eat it all in a few minutes. She said that now one piece seemed to satisfy her for a few days, and it lasted and lasted.

As I have mentioned, most patients are eventually able to eat all the types of food they could eat before their surgery, but there are some exceptions. Some patients have one or two foods that they can't tolerate. Most commonly these include red meat, tomatoes, onions, milk, and ice cream. There are rare patients who claim that they can't tolerate any solid foods, and that they live only on liquids. These patients need a good diagnostic workup, probably including X-rays and endoscopy, because all patients should be able to eat most foods.

Most gastric-bypass patients seem to be happy with their new eating habits. They eat two or three meals a day, and the size of the meals is acceptable to them. They know they are eating as much as they should, and do not regret that they are unable to overeat or gorge themselves. They no longer eat large quantities because they are unhappy. They eat moderately because they are hungry and because they enjoy their food.

As my experience with the gastric bypass in New York increased, the gastric bypass became a routine event. I learned a great deal about the patients and their reaction to the surgery. The results of the surgery, as you will see in chapter 18, were generally good without the long list of complications that I used to see.

18

New York Results

I am a great eater of beef, and I believe that does harm to my wit.
—Shakespeare, *Twelfth Night*

The six hundred patients that I have operated on since moving to New York City are similar in most respects to those in Syracuse. The average patient is thirty-six years old, with a range of fourteen to sixty-five years, although I operated on one patient who was sixty-nine years old. The patients have mostly been women, outnumbering men six to one. My patients come from all walks of life, and have included physicians, lawyers, teachers, nurses, pulmonary therapists, hospital employees, bank employees, real-estate agents, advertising executives, insurance-company employees, restaurant owners, butchers, computer salespeople, jewelers, locksmiths, social workers, civil-service workers, school-bus drivers, policemen, police dispatchers, secretaries, students, laborers, and others. Many of the women were homebound with children. Many of the others were unemployed, some because of physical disabilities.

The average weight of my patients is 297 pounds and the range has been from 179 to 555 pounds. The heights of the patients varied widely, from 4 feet 10 inches to 6 feet $8\frac{1}{2}$ inches, averaging at 5 feet 5 inches. A few have been slightly less than 100 pounds over ideal weight, but have serious medical problems relating to their obesity. Most are well over 100 pounds overweight. Similar to the earlier groups of morbidly obese patients that I had operated on, my New York patients were burdened with obesity-related medical problems. These include high blood pressure, diabetes, back pains, arthritis of the weight-bearing joints, shortness of breath with activity, and others.

WEIGHT LOSS

The surgical results have been good. Overall, the average weight loss has been 36 percent of the starting weight (Fig. 11). The best percentage weight loss was that of the 555-pound patient Charles, whose weight was reduced to 215 pounds when I saw him last, three and a half years after the operation. This was a 61 percent loss. Up until March of 1987, nearly 89 percent of my patients lost at least 25 percent of their weight. Since that time, when we started using the new stapling instrument, 96 percent of patients have lost at least 25 percent. And 99 percent have lost at least 20 percent of their weight.

The weight loss itself is interesting. It seems more dramatic during the first few months, and gradually it slows with each successive month until the weight levels off at about a year after the operation. About 10 percent (8 to 12 percent is the range) of the patient's weight is lost during the first month. We see the weight loss first in the patient's face. This is particularly encouraging for those patients who have full, rounded faces. Then gradually the rest of the body begins to look thinner. Many patients report that their feet get smaller and that their shoe size decreases by as much as two sizes. Breast size also may decrease, which is good for some and not so good for others. Naturally, the patients' waists get smaller, and I usually tell my male patients to save the belts they used before the operation. It makes a good souvenir as well as a reminder of how big they once were.

There are a few other interesting aspects of this weight loss. As I mentioned in chapter 13, much of the fatty tissue just beneath the skin is lost, and the patients start to feel chilly, even in the hottest weather. Also, as this fatty tissue and the weight in general is lost, some patients begin to have sagging and redundant skin. Fortunately, most patients, probably about 80 percent of them, have enough elasticity in the skin for it to shrink down as the weight reduces. But for others, especially the oldest and the heaviest ones, they have so much excess skin that they need plastic surgery. This mainly involves the abdominal wall, but also the arms (sometimes called "bat wings"), thighs, buttocks, breasts, and chin. Some patients wanted "a little of everything done." And some got very vain

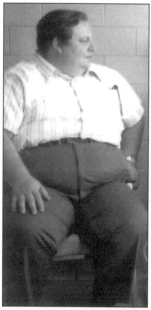 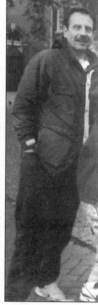

Fig. 11. Patients before and after gastric bypass. (Reproduced by permission of the patients)

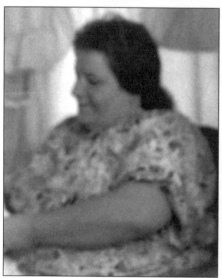 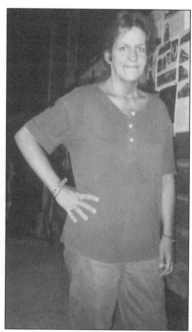

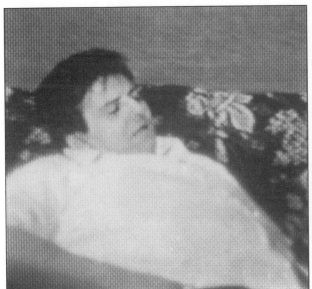
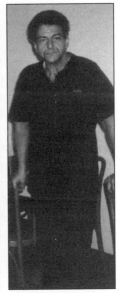
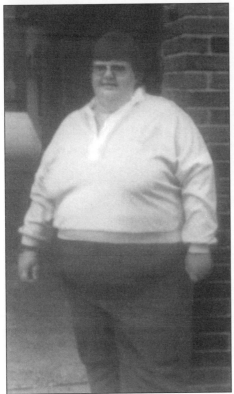
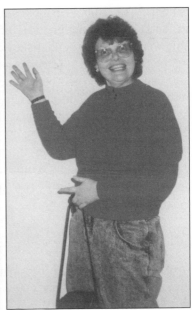

about their appearance. I think that's fine. I was glad to see that they now cared very much how they looked. But we'll talk more about plastic surgery later on.

There's one more strange thing that happened with the loss of weight. Every so often I get a telephone call from a patient who has lost a lot of weight. "Dr. Ackerman, I have a tumor growing out of my surgical incision." I then ask if it's at the top or the bottom of the incision. If it's the bottom, it usually is a small hernia that developed in the incision. The hernia means that the overlying skin is intact, but beneath the skin, the muscle and fibrous layer that I sewed together after completing the operation has separated. When the patient strains the abdomen, a bulging is seen. These hernias mostly occur in the lower part of the incision.

Now, if this "tumor" is in the upper part of the incision, that's a different story. There is a small, fingerlike piece of hard cartilage that we all have attached to the lowest part of the sternum, or breastbone. It's only about an inch long, and isn't very visible. The name of this structure is the *xiphoid*. Most people have never heard of it, but we all have one. Most of us can feel the xiphoid on our bodies if we try. But not the morbidly obese patients. The xiphoid is covered over with a deep layer of fat in these patients, and they are unaware of its existence. When they lose considerable weight, all of a sudden they can feel this "tumor." Often it is actually more apparent than on thinner people because cartilage, even hard cartilage can be moved and bent. Morbidly obese people have increased pressure within their abdominal cavities because of the great amount of fat within. This pressure chronically pushes against the xiphoid which, instead of lying flat, is actually sticking upward on an angle. So when enough weight is lost, the xiphoid is seen and felt, and some patients become concerned about a tumor. At this point, I give the patients a little anatomy lesson, and they learn to live with their "new" xiphoid.

PATIENTS' STORIES

As a result of the weight loss, many of the patients experience major positive changes in their lives. One patient, Daisy, for example, had diabetes, high blood pressure, gallstones, and very disabling arthritis involving her legs. At fifty-two years of age, she had been in a wheelchair for sixteen years. After surgery, her weight dropped from about 370 pounds to 230 pounds, a 38 percent loss. Her diabetes and high blood pressure cleared up, her gallbladder was removed, and of greatest importance to her, she was able to get out of her wheelchair. She still needed a walker to help her get around, but she is now able to shop, cook for her family, and take care of her house.

Another woman, Emily, thirty-four years of age, had been trained as a pulmonary therapist, but was unable to work because of her excessive 320 pounds. When I last heard from her, more than a year after surgery, she weighed 195 pounds, a 40 percent weight loss, and is back at work in pulmonary therapy.

Another patient, Susanna, who had disabling pains in her back and legs experienced a complete disappearance of her symptoms after her weight loss. During one of the postoperative visits, she told me she is painting her house. I asked her, casually, if she is satisfied with the painters. She replied, "You misunderstand me. I'm doing the painting. I'm up on the ladders outside the house doing the work."

Other changes, less dramatic, sometimes occur. One thirty-one-year-old woman, Doris, was an operating-room nurse at one of the hospitals in the city. She had always been given extra shifts and added hours to work because her supervisors felt that at 320 pounds she had no social life to go home to and wouldn't mind working extra hours. She knew that they were taking advantage of her, but she let them "push her around." When she underwent a gastric bypass and her weight dropped to about 200 pounds (a 38 percent loss), a new personality emerged. She is now "tough as nails." She commands a lot more respect, and "They don't dare to push me around anymore!" Was she happier? You bet!

Another patient, Betty, a physician, said that everything was better in her life after her weight loss, including getting married. But there was one concern. Before her weight loss, when she walked down the crowded corridors in her hospital everyone moved aside, out of her way rather than be bumped by her. After the weight loss, the situation changed. She now has to fight her way, as everyone else did, as she walks through the crowds in the corridors, no longer being protected by her former bulk. She also expresses to me a very common problem that people who are no longer morbidly obese experience. It is often very difficult at first for them to realize and to accept the fact that they are no longer obese. This physician, in a clothing store, would immediately head for the oversized section. As she walked on, she would catch a glimpse of herself in a mirror, and then suddenly realize that she no longer needed those sizes, and that she could buy regular clothing off the rack. She also tells me that while sitting in a restaurant with a friend one day, they happened to notice a thin, attractive woman walk by. My patient said to her friend that she wished she looked like that. Her friend, astonished at this comment, replied, "But you do look like that!" My formerly obese patient thought for a moment, and then answered, "That's right, I guess I do."

Other patients have had similar experiences. They have lived for years as very obese, often unattractive individuals, and it is hard for them to realize that this has all changed. Some still associate with their very obese friends, still feeling that they belong with them.

Eventually they accept the existence of their new appearance, and they start to enjoy it. They buy new, often brighter clothes. More attractive makeup is used. And many became more outgoing, emerging from the shadows with a brighter personality.

Just as the patients had difficulties recognizing themselves, others, even friends and relatives, are often unable to recognize their new appearance. I have heard so many stories about this: A patient goes to a family reunion a year after surgery, and no one in the family has any idea who this person is. A patient goes out to dinner with her husband, and she becomes aware that a friend sitting nearby is afraid to come over because she doesn't know who the husband is dining with.

Patients often have the same difficulties with their business associates and customers. One patient, Raymond, a restaurant owner, was visited by one of his suppliers who hadn't seen him for a year. The supplier asked, "Whatever happened to that fat guy who used to own this place?"

Some patients experience situations that almost become serious problems because of their change in appearance. One woman, Elizabeth, was stopped by the police for a minor motor infraction. When asked, she produced her driver's license. This created a problem. In many states, there is a picture of the driver on the license. The police would not believe that this was her license. She looked so different from the picture taken when she was still obese. The patient had to do a lot of fast talking to convince the police that she was indeed the same person, minus many pounds of weight.

Some patients have needed a lot of reassurance from me that they still are going to function as well in their daily routines after they lose the weight. One thirtyish man who was 6 feet 3 inches and 340 pounds was concerned about his ability to continue to play baseball as a recreation. He was an outfielder. I reassured him that his running game and his fielding would probably be improved, but I couldn't be sure about his ability as a long-ball hitter. He had a good weight loss down to the low 200s.

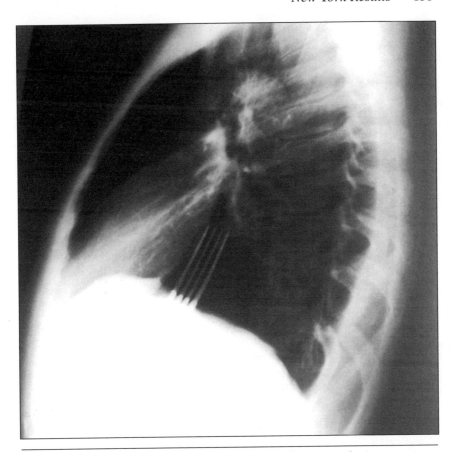

Fig. 12. X-ray showing swallowed fork in gastric-bypass patient.

Happily, as predicted, his running and fielding were better, and even without his extra weight, his hitting ability did not change.

There is one more story I would like to relate. This concerns a forty-two-year-old man, Reginald, whom I operated on when he weighed about 320 pounds. He had an excellent result, and a year after surgery his weight was down to 165 pounds, a 49 percent loss. One day, he was having a late lunch in a restaurant. Some of the food he was eating appeared to get stuck in his throat, and would neither go down nor could he cough it up. He grabbed the nearest implement, a fork, and put it in the back of his throat to push the food down. It worked, and he was relieved. The only problem was that he couldn't find the fork. He assumed it dropped on the floor, but he couldn't find it anywhere. It then dawned on him that he must have swallowed it! He called me, told me the story, and reported that he felt no discomfort or pain. I told him to go immediately to his neighborhood hospital and have them X-ray his chest and abdomen. The fork was there, in his gastric pouch and esophagus (Fig. 12). His gastroenterologist tried removing it using an endoscope put down into the stomach, but felt it was too dangerous. The problem was that the tines were positioned upward, and by pulling out the fork there was a good possibility that the esophagus could be perforated or injured. He needed an operation. An opening was made in the gastric pouch and the fork was removed. Fortunately, he healed well without any complications. I told him, even after losing almost 50 percent of his weight he had to be careful what he put into his mouth.

Many patients, possibly most of them, are nervous and worried about the whole process before the surgery is done. I don't blame them. Most are in reasonably good health except for their obesity, and I am going to put them asleep and cut them up. This is a scary situation. I try to get them to think about their life a year hence, when they will be thinner and healthier. I do not pressure them in any way to have the surgery. They are told emphatically that it is their decision. Sometimes their spouses, parents, and other family members are firmly against the surgery. They themselves are not morbidly obese and really don't understand the situation. "All you have to do is get on a diet, show some self-control, and you'll lose the weight," they say. Even some of their doctors are against the surgery. "Just diet!" they say. If I am asked by the patient what my advice is, I say, "It's your body and your health. You have to decide how best to take care of it." And some patients decide to have the surgery, and others don't.

Many patients have some trouble making up their minds on whether to have the surgery or not. Some just don't show up in the hospital on the day they are supposed to be admitted. A few of these people call me with an excuse which may or may not be real. None of this bothers me. The surgery is elective, and the decision is theirs to make. Occasionally the patient is admitted to the hospital, but leaves the night before the operation after having changed his or her mind. And then the ultimate: I have had five or six patients who actually changed their minds right on the operating table, and got up and walked out. I remember one patient, Barbara, who did this. She was scheduled to have her gastric bypass one day after I performed the same operation on her mother. She was a little stunned to see her mother with all the tubes and IVs going into her, and she thought about this on the operating-room table before being put to sleep. She changed her mind. Everyone in the room, nurses and anesthesiologists, were shocked. That is, everyone but me. I had seen this happen before. I said, "I think she'll be back once her mother gets over the operation." Sure enough, after a few months she had her gastric bypass, and even had a better result than her mother. Most of the patients who walked off the operating table have come back later for the surgery.

IMPROVEMENT IN DIABETES

As the patients lose weight, improvements in their health and their physical disabilities often occur. There are usually major improvements in diabetes, although the mechanisms involved are probably different from those occurring after the intestinal bypasses. With the gastric bypass, changes are more gradual. Abnormal blood sugar levels drop down to normal at an average time of two months after the gastric bypass, although it may take as long as five months. Glucose tolerance tests, where the patient drinks a sweetened sugar solution and has blood glucose levels measured at certain intervals, are often difficult to perform after the gastric bypass. The problem in these postoperative patients is that they are often unable to swallow and retain this very sweet drink. But when the test is successfully performed in these patients, it is usually normal after the operation, even if it is very abnormal before surgery.

At New York Medical College we studied about thirty of our patients who required either daily insulin injections or pills to control their diabetes. Between 80 and 90 percent of these patients were able to discontinue completely all medications, at an average of two to three months after surgery. There were several patients who had their medications discontinued immediately after the operation. The few patients still needing insulin were able to reduce their doses by about 80 percent, and were better controlled. The major reason for this improvement is probably the greatly reduced food intake, particularly the decrease in carbohydrates. The actual weight loss, as it gradually occurred, also played a role in continuing and maintaining this improvement. There may even be other factors.

OTHER IMPROVEMENTS

Most of the other improvements in health that are seen after the gastric bypass are similar to those occurring after the intestinal bypass. Most of the patients who had suffered from high blood pressure were able to decrease or discontinue their medications after surgery. Those patients with breathing problems were also greatly improved. Back and joint pains decreased, sometimes completely, but much depended on the actual status of the joints. Even when the joints were ravaged with destructive changes before surgery, improvement does occur in the months following surgery. Just carrying around less weight decreases the strain on these joints. Blood triglyceride levels decrease as the patient's weight goes down. Cholesterol levels in the blood also drop somewhat, but not so rapidly or so much as after the intestinal bypass.

Psychological and social improvements are seen in the majority of patients. Changes include an increase in self-confidence, and decreases in neurotic tendencies, depression, and hysteria. The quality of life improves. I have known of many patients who returned to school, obtained better jobs, got married, had children, and made significant changes in their lives. I have probably had about twenty patients who became pregnant after the gastric bypass, and all had normal pregnancies, normal deliveries, and normal children.

With the weight loss and the major improvements in some of the obesity-related medical problems, we felt that we had achieved a desirable goal. Patients not only did well, but they were generally pleased with the results. However, as you will see, nothing is perfect. There were complications, although not as frequent and severe as after the intestinal bypasses.

19

Complications and Failures of Gastric Bypass

I cannot eat but little meat,
My stomach is not good.
                —John Still, *Gammer Gurton's Needle*

Nothing's perfect in this life, or at least very few things are. The gastric-bypass operation is no exception, although it is one of the best ways to treat morbid obesity. There are a number of complications that can occur, but most are uncommon, and some are rare. These problems are usually correctable, although sometimes making the diagnosis can be difficult.

As I mentioned earlier, the gastric-bypass operation has often been fairly difficult to perform, and problems could occur during the operation. I also mentioned about injuries to the spleen, although usually I was able to avoid this complication. There could be a moderate amount of bleeding during the operation. As I gained more experience, the amount of blood loss in each operation greatly decreased. We rarely needed to transfuse patients. I had performed this operation on several Jehovah's Witness patients, whose religion forbids them to accept blood transfusions, and there was never a problem.

Immediately after the operation, we worried about the expansion of the lungs and breathing. Patients were told to take deep breaths to expand their lungs fully, and they were taught how to cough without increasing the pain and discomfort in their incisions. This was all very important since it helped to prevent pneumonia and other lung problems. Pulmonary emboli (blood clots to the lungs) were things we worried about since they can be life threatening. We were taught that obese patients had a much higher incidence of this serious complication. But it didn't seem to be so. It was my experience and also the experience of many other surgeons that this complication was rare in our morbidly obese patients. Nevertheless, we did take a lot of precautions to prevent it. Probably the most effective thing we did was the use of compressive boots on the patient during the operation and for several days afterward. These are expandable plastic coverings that are programmed to squeeze the lower legs periodically. This simulated walking or other activity of the legs, and kept the circulation of the veins in the leg active.

INFECTIONS

For me, the most feared complication after surgery is a perforation or leak of the gastrointestinal tract. The perforations theoretically could occur in the gastric pouch, in the lower stomach, or in the jejunum near the connection we made with the gastric pouch. A leak could occur in the suture line where we connected the stomach to the jejunum. There are a number of potential causes for these problems, including distention of the stomach with air after surgery, a "pistol shot perforation" due to pressure from the nasogastric tube, injury, or a decrease in local circulation of the stomach wall, etc.

The diagnosis should be easy since the pouring out of fluid from these organs into the abdominal cavity should cause intense pain and peritonitis. But somehow the patients did not experience this type of discomfort or pain, and physical exam was generally not very helpful. The white cell count was usually elevated in most patients after this operation, so this test was not helpful in determining infection. Neither is the body temperature, even if it became slightly elevated. What was helpful in making us suspicious was the pulse rate if it rose above 120 beats per minute. Also, the patient just didn't look too well, and appeared very anxious. Fortunately, these complications were very uncommon. Also, we were able to diagnose these problems early because the rubber drains that we place in the abdomen allow the fluids leaking from the stomach or intestines to reach the outside of the body. The drains were also the treatment since they provided a pathway for the fluid to get to the outside, preventing the development of internal abscesses and peritonitis. This permitted the stomach or jejunum to heal. Recovery was slow, but most patients did not need further surgery. Again, these were uncommon problems.

Infections in the incisions should theoretically be fairly common, or so we had been taught. Again, the reality was that they were not very common in the experience of most surgeons who do these operations. Managing these infections in the morbidly obese patient was different than in thinner individuals. We were very conservative, and opened only a very small part of the incision to make sure that the infection is able to drain itself out. If we opened up most or all of the incision, as we do in thinner patients, the healing of the incision, even after the infection is cleared up, might take several months.

VOMITING

The only common problem that the patients experience after the gastric bypass was vomiting. In fact, I don't consider vomiting a complication; I call it a side effect of the operation. Only four out of the hundreds of patients I operate on had not vomited. Vomiting was due to several causes. First is the obvious fact that the gastric pouch is small and the outlet (stoma) we make is also small. If the patient eats more than the capacity of the pouch there is only one place the food can go. Out. Fortunately, most patients learn what their capacity is, and vomiting from this cause stops. The second reason for vomiting is that some foods are just not tolerated well at first. I mentioned some of these earlier. There are a lot of individual differences in food tolerance from patient to patient. Eventually, food tolerance improves and the vomiting stops. Sometimes there appear to be emotional problems causing the vomiting, and every so often vomiting seems to be related to coincidental medical problems, such as infections in the gallbladder, kidney, or inner ear.

Sometimes patients complain that certain medicines bring on a bout of vomiting, or make their vomiting worse. The smell and taste of some of the multivitamins are often the culprits. I had one patient who was having a problem with vomiting, and at the advice of a friend, started with a medicine that "you took for vomiting." But she complained that it only seemed to make things worse. I asked what the medicine was. She replied Ipecac®. I shook my head in disbelief, and then explained to her that Ipecac® is indeed used for vomiting. Not for stopping it, but for *inducing* vomiting, in patients who swallowed poison, for example.

When a patient complains of serious vomiting I usually try to find out what the patient is eating, and I make suggestions of foods that might be better tolerated. Also, I sometimes prescribe certain medications that might take the edge off the nausea, such as Compazine® or Tigan®. Reglan®, which improves the functioning of the stomach muscle, is also helpful. If nothing seems to work, I order an X-ray of the stomach, an upper GI series, to see if there is a blockage of the stoma. If I am suspicious of this, I arrange for one of my associates to do endoscopy of the stomach. The endoscope is a tube with a fiberoptic light system, and it is put into the mouth down into the stomach. The endoscopist is able to see into the stomach, and can measure the size of the opening of the stoma. If it is narrowed by scarring or inflammation, the endoscopist is able to thread a small wire in the endoscope through the stoma, and by expanding a small balloon attached to the wire, dilate the stoma enough for the patient to eat without having nausea or vomiting. It's really a remarkable technique. It works on most patients with this problem, and usually one session of dilating is sufficient. Patients go home, and immediately are able to eat. This complication of stomal blockage isn't very common in my experience, but it could occur in a small percentage of patients.

When gastric-bypass patients vomit for any reason, they usually don't become dehydrated because they don't lose stomach or intestinal fluids. They usually lose only what they have eaten. On the other hand, if they experience considerable vomiting for a number of days in a row without holding down anything, they could become very dehydrated and might even need admission to the hospital for replacement of fluids and salts. Again, this is not a very common complication.

Sometimes when the patients have a problem with vomiting they report that they are throwing up bitter greenish, yellowish fluid. This is bile, coming up from the intestines through the stoma into the stomach. This seems to be more common during the first few months after surgery. Often bile bubbles up into their mouths while they are sleeping. Very unpleasant. When this happens, I tell them to elevate the head of the bed about six inches or so, by putting a few books or blocks under the legs of the bed. This simple measure seems to work most of the time. In time, this problem seems to disappear.

GASTROINTESTINAL TRACT PROBLEMS

At first, most patients are constipated, probably because they tend to be dehydrated from the limitation of their liquid intake, and also because they are not eating anything with bulk. Some patients need suppositories or bulking agents added to their diet. But gradually they improve, and their bowel habits return to normal.

In chapter 15 I mention the possibility of developing ulcers after this operation. It is, fortunately, a very uncommon problem, occurring in less than 1 percent of my patients. Also, the ulcers tend to be treatable with antacids and other medications. I had one patient who was resistant to the medications for the ulcer he developed, and he needed an operation to cut the *vagus nerves* near his stomach. These are the nerves that, when stimulated, cause the release of acid in the stomach. The operation was surprisingly easy (he had lost a lot of weight), and his ulcer healed.

Problems that occur late, well after the gastric bypass, are very rare. In fact, when a patient is no longer troubled with vomiting, I usually say, "Now you can enjoy your life," because they are feeling well without problems and are continuing to lose weight.

The one possible exception to the rarity of later problems is the development of gallstones. I say "possible" because there is a major difference of opinion between surgeons as to how often this occurs. In my experience, and in the experience of most surgeons this is fairly uncommon, possibly occurring in about 3 to 6 percent of patients. But some surgeons have reported a much greater incidence. One group of surgeons write that 24 percent of their gastric-bypass patients develop gallstones during the first few years after their surgery. This incidence is so high that they recommend that all morbidly obese patients have their gallbladders removed during the gastric-bypass operation. There are other surgeons who have had similar experience and remove the gallbladders in all their bypass patients. I think, however, that most surgeons only remove it if gallstones are present.

Some neurological complications occur after the gastric bypass, but most of these are very uncommon or even rare. The one complication I saw is something called *meralgia paresthetica*. Patients with this problem complain of burning, tingling, or numbness on the upper outer part of both thighs. It is apparently caused by pressure put on the nerves of the skin in this area. How it actually happens is a little uncertain. It may be due to pressure from the metal retractors we use during the operation to give us good exposure of the operative field, but can also have been due to tight belts used by the patients or even the pressure from the obesity itself. Possibly 10 or 20 percent of the patients have this problem, but in some it is very minimal. Fortunately, it is completely reversible, although it frequently takes from two to six months to disappear completely. It really is not a serious problem.

VITAMIN DEFICIENCIES AND ANEMIA

Vitamin deficiencies and anemia also occur in these patients, but both are generally easily treated. These mostly involve vitamin B_1, vitamin B_{12}, and iron, and respond well to replacement therapy. Iron deficiency may be due to a decrease in absorption in the body, and also to the avoidance by the patient of foods containing iron, particularly beef. For patients needing vitamin replacement, I usually recommend taking the chewable vitamins, especially in the early months after surgery. Later on the capsules are fine.

DEATH

As with any major operation, there is a risk of dying as a result of this operation. We worry about heart attacks, pulmonary emboli (blood clots to the lungs), and major infections. Although these are all uncommon, they can occur, since we are operating on very obese patients. Fortunately, the risks of dying are low, less than 1 percent in many surgeons' experience. And keep in mind that morbid obesity is itself a cause of death in patients who are not operated on. Clearly, the benefits are greater than the risks.

FAILURE TO LOSE WEIGHT

As in any type of surgery, we have had failures. I consider it a failure if the patient doesn't lose at least 25 percent of his or her starting weight. We have had only about 4 percent failures, for which there are two major causes. First, the patient may be taking in excessive calories in spite of the limitations imposed by the stapling, thus defeating the effort at weight loss. Drinking large amounts of high-calorie liquids or frequently eating small amounts of high-calorie foods could cause this. Sometimes discussing this with the patient improved the situation, with the patient switching to a low-calorie liquid. But at other times, the patient has already gained much of the weight back, and there is little that could be done.

I operated on one young woman, Roberta, who did very well for the first several months after her surgery. But long before the first postoperative year had arrived, she started to regain weight. I became very concerned, and tried to find out what was going wrong. After much discussion, I found out why. She spent her days at home with her small children. All day long she walked around the house carrying a glass of one of the popular cola sodas. Not diet soda, of course. She never drank enough at one time to fill up her stomach and feel full. Instead, she sipped on the soda. And sipped and sipped. All day long. As the glass gradually emptied, she refilled it, and sipped some more. She admitted that in an average day, she finished three liter bottles of soda! And that was in addition to her regular, small meals. I figured that her soda added about 1,300 calories to her daily intake. No wonder she gained weight. Fortunately, in her case, we managed to convince her to switch over to a diet soda, and she lost the weight again.

The second reason for failure is related to a technical problem from the operation. The most common problem used to be the pulling apart of some of the staples so that the staple line was no longer completely intact. As a result, all of a sudden the patient was able to eat as much as before the operation, and the pounds would start mounting. With the new stapling instrument, this problem greatly decreased in frequency. There still are the two other technical problems, the enlarging of the connection between the stomach and intestine, and the stretching of the upper stomach.

Whenever I have a patient whose weight loss is inadequate, or whose weight is starting to rise significantly after a good weight loss, I try to find out several things. What are they eating? How many meals per day? Is there snacking and on what types of foods? How soon after eating does the patient get hungry again? I usually get an X-ray of the stomach, an upper GI series (Figs. 13–16). If there is any suggestion of staples pulling apart, enlargement of the stoma, or stretching of the pouch, I consider a reoperation. The X-rays aren't perfect, but frequently they give me a hint of a technical problem.

I really don't like doing the reoperations, but as I told the patients, I don't like failures either. The problem with the reoperations is the adhesions that most, but not all patients develop after the original operation. Everything is stuck together, particularly the stomach and the liver. Separating these organs from each other is tedious and difficult, and has to be done carefully to avoid injury. As soon as the stomach and intestine are freed from the adhesions, I try to find out what the problems are. You can't

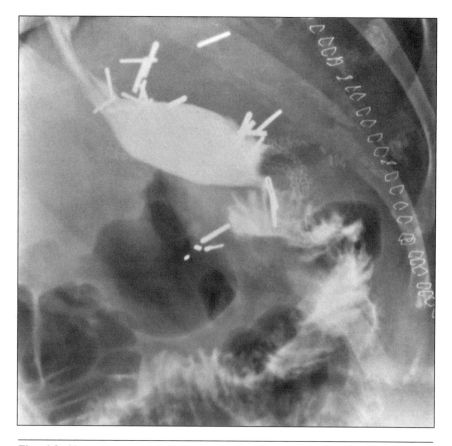

Fig. 13. Normal appearance of upper GI series after gastric bypass. (Dye in small gastric pouch slowly empties into the intestine.) (Reprinted by permission, *Gastrointestinal Surgery* 2 [1985])

see the stomach staples since they are well buried in the stomach wall. But you can feel if there are gaps in the staple line that would allow food to go into the lower stomach. The stoma between the stomach and intestine can be felt and the opening can be measured with a ruler. The size of the gastric pouch is examined, and in my mind I compare it to what it looked like at the original operation.

The final step is to correct the problem. If it is the staple line, I restaple the stomach using the new stapling instrument. If the problem is enlargement of the pouch, I remove some of the excess stomach in the area between the stoma and the esophagus on the upper left side of the pouch.

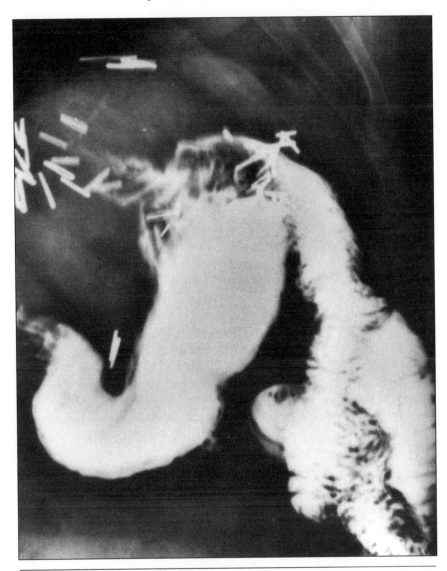

Fig. 14. Disruption of staples. (Dye goes from the small gastric pouch directly into the rest of the stomach, as well as into the intestine.) (Reproduced by permission from *General Surgery 2,* revised edition, edited by John J. Byrne, M.D., and Harry S. Goldsmith, M.D. [Philadelphia: Harper & Row, 1984])

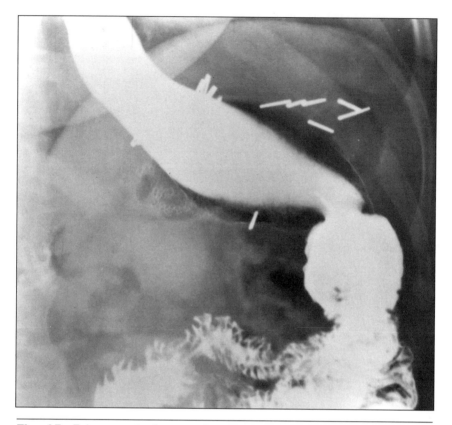

Fig. 15. Enlargement of stoma between the stomach and the intestine. (Reprinted by permission, *Gastrointestinal Surgery* 2 [1985])

Narrowing the size of the stoma is more difficult. The first technique I use is to put stitches at right angles to the opening to try to close it down partially. This works on a short-term basis, but there are failures that can occur. Later I use a row of staples placed completely across the stoma, but first I remove six individual staples in the middle of the row. Removing these staples leaves a small opening between the stomach and intestine, in the range of 8 to 10 millimeters. This technique seems to be better.

Patients seem to tolerate the second operation better than the first. One of the reasons is that less is done during this operation, and it often is a shorter operation. Another reason is that patients already know what to expect after this type of operation, and there are no unpleasant surprises.

The results after these reoperations are variable. The least that hap-

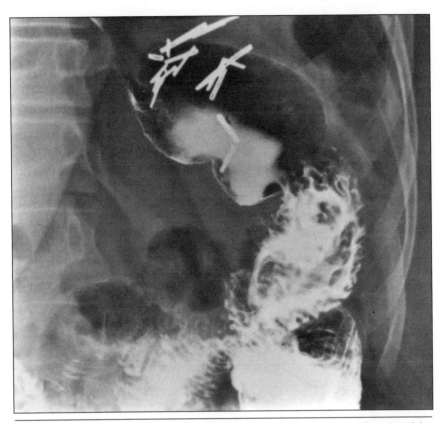

Fig. 16. Enlargement of gastric pouch after gastric bypass. (Reprinted by permission, *Gastrointestinal Surgery* 2 [1985])

pens is that regaining of further weight stops cold. At best, there is a very significant weight loss, sometimes more than after the original operation. Most patients experience some weight loss, especially during the first few months. Frequently, a small weight loss after the second operation coupled with some weight loss remaining after the first procedure adds up to a satisfactory result.

I've tried to give all the various negatives about the gastric bypass, but even with all this, I feel that the gastric bypass is the best answer we have to the serious problem of morbid obesity.

20

Morbid Obesity in
Teenagers and Grandparents

> I was resolved to grow fat and look young till forty.
> —John Dryden, *The Maiden Queen*

Most of the patients I have operated on have been between twenty and fifty years old, with an average age of about thirty-four years. But there have been some young ones, in their teens, and also some relatively elderly ones, over fifty-five years of age. I find these groups of patients to be particularly interesting.

TEENAGERS

There have been a few articles in the surgical journals written about the use of these weight-reducing operations in young people. As I recall, the youngest patient mentioned was an eleven-year-old. Results, with the intestinal bypass in the earliest paper, and with the gastric bypass in later papers were generally good, except for children with the *Prader-Willi syndrome* which we'll discuss in chapter 21.

The youngest potential patient I ever saw was six years old! One of our surgeons at New York Medical College asked me to see this boy and his family. I was very reluctant to think about this, because my feeling has been that these operations should only be done on patients who have reached adult growth and height. I am just not sure what the effect of the very restricted food intake would be on actual growth. But I did agree to meet with the boy, Billy, and his family, at least to talk. At six years of age he weighed 150 pounds. No doubt about it, he was very obese. But the family situation disturbed me very much. The tension in the air between the mother and father was obvious from the start. The father finally walked out after a short while, mumbling that he didn't want to be a part of any of this. The boy appeared to take great delight in the whole proceedings. Every time the mother mentioned how much he eats, how much he weighs, and how big he was, the boy reacted positively. A big smile spread across his face. He appeared to enjoy the attention he was getting from his mother, and from all of us. I felt this whole situation was not healthy, and suggested that family counseling would be the route for them to go. Certainly not a gastric bypass on this six-year-old.

I have operated on teenagers, probably more than twenty of them through the years. All of them were big and fully grown. Their preoperative weights ranged from about 228 pounds in a 5 foot 4 inch nineteen-year-old girl to about 510 pounds in a 6 foot 0 inch tall eighteen-year-old boy. Most weighed between the high 200s to the mid-300s, with the average being about 305 pounds. All were over 5 feet tall, with most boys between 5 feet 7 inches to 6 feet 1 inch. Surprisingly, the girls barely outnumbered the boys, less than two to one. The very youngest patient was a fourteen-year-old boy who weighed about 345 pounds.

My first experience with the teenagers was with the intestinal bypass. I operated on four patients, weighing from 300 to 510 pounds. The results were exceptionally good. The weight losses varied from 42 to 58 percent. One nineteen-year-old male, Arnie, went from 470 pounds to 195 pounds. The heaviest patient, Vic, dropped his weight from about 510 to 284 pounds, which at a height of six he carried well. He had had severely bowed legs from early childhood which greatly limited his ability to walk and run. I heard that after his weight loss he was able to have successful corrective surgery done on his deformed legs.

The rest of my experience with the teenage group involved the gastric-bypass operation. These kids were treated the same as my older patients. The operation was the same, as well as the postoperative care. And the results were the same as our adult patients, with an average 36 percent weight loss of those who were followed for at least twelve months. Some of these teenagers did not keep their postoperative appointments. I thought this was strange. Most came to see me for the first time with their parents, and the parents were usually present when the operation was performed. So the parents appeared to be concerned about their children's well-being. But for some reason some of the teenagers and their parents did not come back to see me after the first or second post-operative visit. I really don't understand this. I hope the reason was that they were doing so well they felt they didn't need me.

Some of these teenagers were members of families in which excessive obesity was rampant. There were two sisters whose mother I had operated on, two brothers, a brother and sister, and one boy whose mother I had as a patient. In general, the various members of these families had similar results from the surgery. It would have been terrible if one had a good result and the other sibling didn't.

The boys were interesting. Most were active, even athletic, in spite of their weight. Lenny was a first baseman on his Little League team, and his greatest concern was his ability to play ball after the surgery. I told him the obvious, that he would probably not present as big a target for his teammates to throw at, at first base, but that such things as base running should be better. I never did find out how he fared in his baseball. Another 300-pound teenager played on his high school football team. He was a lineman, obviously. I assured him that even after the expected weight loss he would still be big enough to be a lineman.

The girls were another matter. I did not get the feeling, as a group, that they were a particularly active bunch. After they lost weight, most became considerably more attractive. I know of one seventeen-year-old, Frances, whose weight dropped from about 240 to 140 pounds who got married a year or two later. Another girl, Agatha, fifteen years old when she was operated on, lost much weight but was still fairly heavy. This apparently didn't stop her. She became pregnant, had her baby, and then became pregnant again.

Many of these girls had missed out on the fun of being a teenager. It was a great source of satisfaction to me to see them emerge from their restricted lives to begin to take part in the regular activities of their peers. One sixteen-year-old girl, Naomi, 5 feet 9 inches, dropped her weight from 265 to 175 pounds. She really looked good, and became a "regular" teenager. One can just imagine the changes that occurred in her life. That's probably the best part of operating on these young patients. When the weight loss is satisfactory, a person's whole life turns around. These kids can for the first time begin to lead a "normal" life, for all the years to come.

GRANDPARENTS

The older patients are a different story. Much of their lives are already behind them, and many have been unhappy and handicapped for years. Is it worthwhile operating on them? Years ago, the age limit for this type of surgery was fifty, then up to fifty-five years of age. Some surgeons feel that the results in patients over fifty-five are not as good as in younger patients, and that the risks are greater.

I gradually raised the age limit, particularly when I saw that the results were satisfactory, and the benefits were tangible. Many of these patients had developed problems in their backs and legs, and their activity was quite limited. Weight loss appeared to make a major difference in their ability to move and get around. One fifty-five-year-old, Ruth, who had lost considerable weight through surgery, waved her finger at me saying, "Don't you ever again say that you won't operate on a patient over fifty-five. We have some years left to live, and we want to live them in comfort and ease!"

I have now operated on about ten patients who were fifty-five years and older. All were gastric bypasses. Almost all of the patients are females. Their weights were similar to my other patients, ranging from about 250 to 400 pounds. All were reasonably good operative risks for surgery, with no recent heart attacks, and there were no deaths. In fact, the complication rate was low. There were some failures in terms of results. One or two patients had a disruption of their line of gastric staples, but did not want a second restapling operation. The average weight loss of these older patients was just under 30 percent, so possibly they don't do quite as well as the younger patients. The number of patients is small, so this may not be a real statistic difference.

But the weight loss is meaningful to most of these patients. Most of those with arthritic problems have been able to get around much more easily than before. Several have gone back to work, including some who hadn't been able to work for years. Some were able to continue at their employment, but with greater ease. I think the benefits to these people have greatly outweighed the risks, and at the present time my age limit has risen to sixty-five years.

Having said this, I now have to talk about possible exceptions. I was called by a sixty-nine-year-old woman, Clara, who wanted information about the gastric-bypass operation. I told her that my age limit was sixty-five. She stopped me by saying that she was becoming increasingly crippled by the effects of her obesity on her arthritis. She said she was healthy otherwise, and did not want to continue her life as a near-cripple, limited in activity only to her apartment. The possible risks of surgery were acceptable to her, particularly if she had a chance to lose a significant amount of weight.

Well, these days it isn't easy to make exceptions to rules, even if they are one's own self-imposed rules. Someone is looking over your shoulder: insurance companies, lawyers, hospital committees, administrators, the state, the federal government, everyone. I'm not paranoid, just realistic! I was advised by the so-called quality assurance administrators at the hospital to make sure the woman was a very good operative risk, and to write on the hospital chart that she, as an exception to my age limits, was being operated on for the various reasons. Her heart and lungs were checked carefully, and I performed a gastric bypass. She came through beautifully, without problems.

She lost about 100 pounds. Most important, she is considerably more mobile, walking with just a cane. In fact every time I see her she appears to be doing better and better. She subsequently had a plastic surgery procedure, a *panniculectomy*, to remove a large abdominal flap. No longer is she a crippled shut-in.

I am sure there is an upper limit of age for these operations. But much depends on the individual patient, the likely medical and physical problems, overall health, and the possible benefit from the loss of weight.

On the lower end of the age spectrum, I still think these operations should be restricted to those young people who have achieved adult growth and height. But how about, say, a twelve-year-old who is 5 feet 8 inches and weighs 350 pounds? . . .

21

Prader-Willi and Other Syndromes

The first in banquets, but the last in fight.
—Homer, *Iliad*

Ask your family physician about the Prader-Willi syndrome, a compulsive eating disorder, and the chances are good that he or she has never heard of it. Most of my surgical friends and my surgical residents had never heard of it either. This is understandable since there are a great number of diseases or syndromes that are rare, or relatively newly discovered that have not made the headlines in newspapers or in medical journals. I have heard of this syndrome, and have treated a patient because one of its features is extreme obesity.

PRADER-WILLI SYNDROME

It is one of the most interesting causes of morbid obesity, and the patients with Prader-Willi syndrome are fascinating. This condition was first described in 1956 by Drs. Prader, Willi, and associates. Nobody knows exactly how prevalent this syndrome is, but there have been at least six hundred patients identified, and the true incidence is probably many times that number. There is even a Prader-Willi Syndrome Association.

The cause of this syndrome is probably related to genetic or chromosomal defects, at least that seems to be the prevailing opinion. There may actually be some signs of this condition when a fetus is still in the

175

mother's uterus, particularly a decrease in the baby's movements. When the baby is born, there may be some difficulties in feeding and some babies have been fed by tubes or droppers. This may be related to a weakness in muscle strength that occurs in many of these children.

The feeding problems in infancy are ironic, because after a few years it becomes obvious that obesity is becoming a major problem for the child. Other symptoms start to become apparent, such as shortness of stature and some degree of mental retardation. But the precise diagnosis of Prader-Willi is frequently not made until late childhood or even in adulthood.

Most of these patients are short. The average height in one group of these patients was fifty-nine inches for the females, and sixty-one inches for the males. They usually have small hands and feet. Sexual development is retarded in both males and females. The mental retardation is variable, and some patients are only minimally retarded. There are other important findings, but these vary from patient to patient.

Personality problems with wide fluctuations of behavior are common. Temper tantrums often occur, particularly when food is withheld from them, but can occur at other times. They may become manipulative, deceitful, and conniving, and very stubborn. With uncontrollable anger, some of these patients have been hospitalized in locked mental wards. But these outbursts are usually short-lived, and for much of the time the patients are in full control of their emotions.

The obesity is what makes them so very interesting. They start to eat "well" in early childhood, and the weight starts to rise, and rise. Ordinary attempts to control the weight fail. It soon becomes obvious that the obesity is a major problem for them. Their ability to eat is legendary. They eat everything, according to Bray and associates[1] and Zollweger.[2] Cases have been described where Prader-Willi children have eaten dog food and garbage. And the amounts are incredible. But strangely enough, vomiting is extremely rare. Some patients apparently never vomit, even with massive overeating. My patient said that he never experienced the feeling of fullness with his eating.

In one group of patients, the average caloric intake was more than 5,000 calories per day, according to Bray et al.[3] Families of these patients learn to lock food cabinets and refrigerators. In an account in the *New York Times*,[4] the mother forgot to lock the refrigerator when she went out of the house, in spite of her habit of doing so for many years. During her absence, her daughter had eaten the top two inches of a gallon pot of chicken soup, including the congealed fat, four or five pudding pops from the freezer, and several scoops of peanut butter. In another newspaper account, the child managed to lock the mother out of the house, and ate everything on the cupboard shelves.

As you'd expect, the patients with this condition tend to get heavier and heavier, often well into the 300-pound range, and some of the complications of morbid obesity begin to plague them. Diabetes may occur, as well as high blood pressure, breathing problems, and heart disease. I have not seen any reference to what the average life expectancy is, but I know there have been some deaths of fairly young adults with this syndrome. Causes of these deaths are just what you'd expect: heart attacks, pneumonia, and diabetes. In addition to all this, life for other members of the family becomes a living hell.

There does not seem to be any accepted treatment for the syndrome itself, so we're back to diets and surgery. But this is even a more difficult problem than ordinary morbid obesity. All sorts of diets have been tried, and some have had limited success in keeping the weight under a degree of control, particularly if a major effort is made to prevent the massive overeating that can occur. In other words, lock the cabinets, lock the refrigerator, keep the food in the house to a minimum. But even with all this, the failure rate is high.

Surgical procedures have been tried on these Prader-Willi patients. Some of the patients had intestinal bypasses, including an eleven-year-old with the syndrome. Not surprisingly, the expected complications of this operation often occur, and more recent operative experiences have been with gastric-bypass procedures. There have been several reports by Soper and associates,[5] Dietz and Tepper,[6] and Anderson, Soper, and Scott[7] of the effects of gastric bypass on these patients. Weight loss is usually not as great as in non-Prader-Willi patients, and the Prader-Willi patients often stopped losing weight after just a few months. Disruption of the staple line was common. Some of the patients gradually regained much of their lost weight. Still, there were some fairly good results.

MY EXPERIENCE

I have had one patient with this syndrome, and I should say from the start that I have a very positive feeling about him. His story, I think, is a very interesting one. Bruce had a typical Prader-Willi childhood, with a history of poor feeding during the first year of life. Thereafter, his weight started to rise dramatically, and at age fourteen, he weighed 196 pounds. He underwent one of the gastroplasty operations, and a month and a half later he weighed 175 pounds. As time went on, he began to gain back the weight, and it appeared that the gastroplasty stoma had stretched enough for the operation to fail. At age twenty, his weight had climbed to 316 pounds and his height was just 5 feet 3 inches. As a result, he developed diabetes and high blood pressure. In spite of appropriate medication, control of the diabetes was not effective. And he had considerable trouble sticking to his diet.

He was given an appointment to see me, but he was skeptical about the benefits of another operation, and was concerned about his chances of survival. I felt he was a good operative risk, and tried to reassure him. He finally asked me if I would sign a statement guaranteeing that he would survive the operation. Now of course this is something no surgeon can do. But I did it for him just to see what his reaction would be. I wrote it out, signed it, and handed it to him. I asked him what he was going to do with it. He paused for a moment and thought about it. He suddenly realized that if he survived, he didn't need the paper, and if he didn't survive, there was nothing he could do with it anyway. He started laughing. In spite of his syndrome, he had a good sense of humor. (He then tore up my signed statement.)

I was not really sure what to do at his operation. I was afraid he would overeat and disrupt the staples, so I divided the stomach after putting extra rows of staples in and separated the upper and lower parts of the stomach. Then I put heavy silk stitches in to reinforce the lines of staples. Then I started to worry that he might still burst the staple line, and food would get into the abdominal cavity causing peritonitis. So I then stitched the two parts of the stomach against each other, hoping that if he did burst the staple line the food would go into the lower stomach part, and not into the abdominal cavity.

He tolerated the operation very well. One month later his weight was down to 278 pounds and for the first time in his life he felt full when eating and was not always able to drink the full three ounces of liquids. When he ate too much he vomited! By four months after surgery his diabetes disappeared and his blood pressure returned to normal. His weight reached a low point of 238 pounds at eight months. His self-confidence improved, he exercised and was getting tutored.

At eleven months after surgery, he started to gain some weight. It reached 282 pounds within seventeen months after his operation. An

X-ray of the stomach showed an opening in the staple line, as I feared, and it opened into the lower part of the stomach. There was no peritonitis, but the surgery had failed. Back to the drawing board.

I reoperated later that month with the approval of the patient and his mother. But in the operating room, the anesthesia doctors had some trouble getting the IV in his veins, and the patient started a classic temper tantrum. "Dr. Ackerman, get me out of here! Get me out of here!" The nurses looked at me to see what I would do. I'm sure they felt I was some sort of monster. The anesthesia doctors whispered to me, "What should we do?" The patient yelled further, "Get me out of here!" I whispered to the anesthesiologists, "Put him to sleep." They asked me again, "What should we do?" I then yelled at them, "Damn it, put him to sleep, now!" Once he was asleep, I explained that this type of outburst was part of his condition, and that both he and his mother definitely wanted the operation to be done. I hope I convinced them, but that was the truth. That was the Prader-Willi syndrome revealing itself. (The patient apologized to me later.)

I did the same operative procedure to begin with, dividing the upper and lower parts of the stomach between the staple lines. But then I placed the *omentum* (a thick pad of fat within the abdominal cavity) between the upper and lower parts of the stomach. This was to act as a barrier between the two parts, so that if the staple line again opened, food would not be able to get into the lower part of the stomach. This operation appears to have worked.

His weight dropped down to between the 230s and the 250s, and remained at this level. He was certainly not even close to an ideal weight, but on the other hand, the diabetes and high blood pressure were gone, and his weight was not increasing. A partial success is sometimes all one can hope for.

He was briefly hospitalized a few years ago for some abdominal pain which quickly disappeared. An X-ray of his stomach at that time showed that the staples were still intact, and everything looked good. But he still had eating and emotional problems.

But I give the young man much credit. He has tried to live as normal a life as possible. He started to take courses at the local community college, but his occasional temper outbursts and his eating behavior in the school cafeteria forced him to stop. Private tutoring by the college was then planned. He was also trying to start vocational training. I know he would like to learn about computers. The last I heard, he was still living on his own. I'm rooting for him to succeed.

OTHER SYNDROMES

There are some other syndromes occurring in children and young people that count obesity among their other medical problems. Some of these are related to over- or underproduction of hormones. Most common is *hypothyroidism*, which is the underproduction of the thyroid hormones. Much less common are syndromes involving the adrenal glands, such as *Cushing's syndrome* (the overproduction of cortisol), and overproduction of androgens (male hormones). But usually, the degree of obesity is not quite so high as to be classified as morbid.

Some other rare syndromes that involve obesity are not related to changes in hormone production. The causes of most of these syndromes are not known, though they may be hereditary or genetic. I'll admit to not being very knowledgeable about these, but I have seen a patient with one of these conditions. One syndrome is called *Laurence-Moon-Biedl*, or *Bardet-Biedl*, or *Laurence-Moon-Bardet-Biedl*, named after the doctors who described the various parts of this condition. Its first descriptions go back over a hundred years. Now, the various components of this syndrome include *retinitis pigmentosa* (deposits of pigment in the retina leading to progressive loss of vision), webbing of the fingers or extra fingers, retarded sexual development, some mental retardation, and obesity, but individual patients may have other medical problems such as congenital heart disease and kidney disease. The syndrome is a bit of a mixture, since patients so afflicted may have some of the features but not necessarily all. The major cause of death in these patients has been related to the kidney disease, although kidney transplantation has certainly improved the outlook. This syndrome can be present in several or many members of a family. Which brings me to the patient I saw several years ago.

This young woman, Angela, about twenty years of age, had the Bardet syndrome, as did her brothers. She was over 300 pounds, but did not have evidence of any mental retardation. Unfortunately, the predominant feature of this condition that ran in her family was severe kidney disease. I believe all of them, including my patient, already had kidney transplants, with varying levels of success. My patient seemed to be doing very well with her new kidney, but she still had the major problem with her weight. When I saw her several years ago she was still taking a great number of medications, mostly to protect her new kidney against rejection. But she was also taking medications for high blood pressure and diabetes. These additional medical problems were probably related to her morbid obesity, and possibly to her transplant.

Weight loss obviously would have been of great benefit to her. The problem was that many of her antirejection medications also tend to interfere with the healing of body tissues. Our fear was that her incision might not heal well, and even more importantly, that the connection we make between the stomach and the intestine might not heal normally. This could be a very dangerous situation. We therefore decided to delay any surgery for her obesity. The hope was that the doses of these medications could be reduced, and the medications finally discontinued. At that point gastric bypass could possibly be reconsidered. The situation is really very sad. She seemed to be a very nice, pleasant young woman who has gone through many difficult years, with multiple operations, many hospitalizations, taking a great deal of medication, and still having problems. She had personal goals in her life, including the desire to attend nursing school. I hope somehow she is able to realize her goals.

I found the Prader-Willi and other syndromes to be very interesting ones. However, they are all very rare. This is probably all for the good, since I am not sure we had a completely successful answer, particularly for the Prader-Willi problem. But there is another syndrome, the Pickwickian syndrome, that is certainly more common, and I think the surgery has been more successful.

NOTES

1. G. A. Bray et al., "The Prader-Willi Syndrome: A Study of Forty Patients and a Review of the Literature," *Medicine* 62 (1983): 59–80.

2. H. Zollweger, "The Prader-Willi Syndrome," *JAMA* 251 (1984): 1835.

3. Bray, "The Prader-Willi Syndrome."

4. D. Clendinen, "Help Sought for Young Victims of Compulsive Eating Disorder," *New York Times*, July 30, 1985.

5. R. T. Soper et al., "Gastric Bypass for Morbid Obesity in Children and Adolescents," *Journal of Pediatric Surgery* 10 (1975): 51–58.

6. W. H. Dietz and D. Tepper, "Surgery for Adolescent and Prader-Willi (P-W) Obesity" (paper presented at the Fourth International Congress on Obesity).

7. A. E. Anderson, R. T. Soper, and D. H. Scott, "Gastric Bypass for Morbid Obesity in Children and Adolescents," *Journal of Pediatric Surgery* 15 (1980): 876–81.

22

Pickwickian Syndrome

> He's fat and scant of breath.
>> —Shakespeare, *Hamlet*

We are all well aware of the interactions between nature and art. The description of Joe the Fat Boy by Charles Dickens in his novel *The Pickwick Papers* (or more accurately *The Posthumous Papers of the Pickwick Club*) must have been based on a real person whom Dickens had seen firsthand. He could not have made it up. It just too accurately describes the appearance of patients with the condition sometimes now called the *Pickwickian syndrome*. Let me quote from Dickens.

"Very extraordinary boy, that," said Mr. Pickwick, "does he always sleep in this way?"

"Sleep!" said the old gentleman, "he's always asleep. Goes on errands fast asleep, and snores as he waits at table."

"How very odd!" said Mr. Pickwick.

"Ah! odd indeed," returned the old gentleman; "I'm proud of that boy—wouldn't part with him on any account—he's a natural curiosity!"

Dickens refers to him as a "fat and red-faced boy," and sometimes calls him "Young Dropsey," "Young Opium-Eater," and "Young Boa Constrictor" in view of his obesity, sleepiness, and enormous appetite.

PICKWICKIAN SYNDROME

This really sums up the appearance of those patients with this Pickwickian syndrome: they are morbidly obese; they sleep, often at inappropriate times; and they are red-faced with a ruddy complexion. Some additional factors must be added that are not so obvious. These patients tend to retain carbon dioxide in their blood, and have a relatively low blood level of oxygen. Sometimes they develop *cyanosis*, or a bluish coloring of the skin from the changes in carbon dioxide and oxygen levels. There may be an increase in the number of red blood cells with thicker, more concentrated blood resulting. They may have respiratory difficulties, and may develop enlargement and failure of the right side of the heart. This is really a very dangerous, even lethal complication of morbid obesity.

Some of these patients also have *sleep apnea*, a disturbance of the normal sleeping pattern at night, with periods of more than ten seconds when the patient makes no effort to breath or has difficulty moving air into his lungs because of airway obstruction. There may be restless awakenings, and periods of very loud snoring. These episodes may occur hundreds of times during the night.

The purists (I am not one) dislike the term Pickwickian syndrome. First of all, they argue, Joe the Fat Boy was not a member of the Pickwickian Club, which was founded by Samuel Pickwick, and that the name Pickwickian should only refer to actual members of the club. Second, they argue, Dickens's description does not include the sleep apnea aspect of the condition, which does occur in many of the patients with this syndrome. So other names have been substituted, most prominently the Obesity-Hypoventilation syndrome. This latter name is satisfactory and accurate, but I really like the term Pickwickian syndrome, because it honors Charles Dickens's powers of observation and description.

The great Canadian physician William Osler had read the novel and suggested in the early 1900s that the term Pickwickian be used to refer to people who are obese and somnolent. But it wasn't until the mid-1950s that morbidly obese individuals with these symptoms were first identified as a specific group.

The syndrome isn't a very common condition. Possibly only as many as 3 to 5 percent of morbidly obese patients have it. And it isn't necessarily the most obese patients that have it. I have seen about a dozen patients with the Pickwickian syndrome, and they have ranged in weight from about 290 to 556 pounds. But the average weight of 370 pounds in this group is higher than that of my total morbidly obese group, and the average age of thirty-nine is also a little older. In my experience, it's more common in males, by about 2 to 1. It apparently can occur in younger patients (my youngest was nineteen years of age). But I have seen a report in a surgical journal of a five-year-old with this problem, and also of a thirty-month-old who was labeled morbidly obese with the obese hypoventilation syndrome requiring mechanical support of her breathing.

My Experience

Sometimes the diagnosis can be made the same way Dickens did. One patient came to see me in one of my group sessions with five other patients. While I was talking about these operations he fell asleep, lightly snoring. The other patients were disgusted, even outraged. They poked him to wake him up, but he just fell asleep again. I told them to leave him alone, explaining that he had this problem associated with his obesity. Another patient in his twenties came in to see me with his parents. As he fell asleep and snored (loudly), the parents were embarrassed, angry at him, and completely disgusted. Again I explained that this was part of the problem. (They never came back to see me again, and he was never operated on, and later I heard that he had died suddenly.) This inappropriate sleeping can occur at any time, while talking, watching television, driving a car, working, eating, and so on.

Other patients first came to my attention by their emergency admissions to the hospital in respiratory failure. Typically they were sleepy, hard to rouse, and almost in coma. Their skin was bluish or cyanotic, and when measured, their blood oxygen level was lower than their carbon dioxide level. An endotracheal tube was placed in their throats and breathing was assisted mechanically. With appropriate medications and breathing support they improved, and the endotracheal tube was eventually removed. At that point, while they were in their best possible condition, I would take them into the operating room and do an antiobesity operation, intestinal bypass in the first few patients, and gastric bypass for the more recent ones.

Some of the patients who were not in acute pulmonary distress underwent formal sleep apnea studies. In these tests, breathing patterns are observed while sleeping, and the presence of these sleep apnea episodes is documented.

In my experience, the patients did amazingly well during the operation, even in spite of their residual breathing problems, and their less than normal pulmonary function. Of course, the anesthesia doctors watched the patients with extra caution. After the operation, the endotracheal tube used for control of breathing during the procedure was left in place, and patients were cared for in the Surgical Intensive Care Unit. Fortunately, after several days the breathing had improved enough to discontinue the mechanical breathing support, and the endotracheal tube could be removed. In one patient the tube was removed after only one day.

I mentioned earlier that this is a very dangerous condition. If not treated adequately, the patients continue to have attacks of breathing problems, and their lungs and hearts get worse. Many eventually die. Some die suddenly and unexpectedly, probably as a result of the breathing problems. Death may be due to a gradual worsening of pulmonary function, even with mechanical support of the lungs. Some patients develop blood clots in their leg veins, and when the clots break lose and travel to the vessels of the lungs death can occur. Heart failure and acute heart attacks are common, and kidney failure can also cause death in these patients. Finally, the falling asleep at inappropriate times can become dangerous. I have heard of patients with this condition who have fallen asleep while driving their cars on highways, crashed, and were seriously injured or died. Is there really any hope for them?

Yes. Weight loss from dieting, an operation, or under any circumstance can reverse the condition, and actually be lifesaving (except when the condition has gone too far and the damage to the heart and lungs has reached an irreversible state). But for most patients with the Pickwickian syndrome weight loss rapidly begins to eliminate their problems. As the weight goes down, the level of oxygen dissolved in their blood rises, and carbon dioxide decreases. Daytime sleepiness disappears and sleep at night gets better. In short, they revert to normal.

Let me tell you about some of my patients. One patient, Myron, offered visual proof of the success from surgery. He was a smoker, which is one of the worst things a Pickwickian can do (besides overeating). And he always dangled his cigarette from the left side of his mouth. He frequently fell asleep while smoking. As a result, all of his shirts and pajama tops had multiple small holes from cigarette burns, all on the left side. I performed an intestinal bypass, and his recovery was difficult during the early postoperative period. But he lost weight and improved significantly. One day, a number of months after his operation he came to see me. He said to me, "Look at my shirt, Dr. Ackerman. You cured me!" Sure enough, his nice new shirt had no holes on the left side. The obvious point was that he no longer fell asleep while smoking, and that the somnolence was gone. (Yes, he did continue to smoke.)

Another patient, Laura, illustrates the need for attacking this condition with early and effective weight loss. She had had several episodes of pulmonary failure. Treatment on two occasions consisted of a tracheotomy which did make her breathing easier. As a result of the inadequate oxygenation of her blood during the periods of respiratory failure, she developed some loss of memory of recent events. For example, in the hospital she was not really sure where she was, so a sign was placed over her bed informing her "You are in the hospital in Syracuse." When I went in to see her for the first time, I introduced myself and told her why I was seeing her. I came back about ten minutes later, and she said, "Do I know you? Have I ever seen you before?" She had forgotten. She did get to know me, and was able to remember who I was. But even after the gastric bypass and its resulting weight loss she never fully recovered her memory. One day she told me that she suddenly started to remember her Social Security number. But gaps in her memory remained as a result of the earlier damage from the breathing problems.

One of the most recent Pickwickian patients I treated, Axel, was referred to me from the Pulmonary Service in the hospital. They realized that his disease was progressing, and that at 433 pounds his prospects were not good. At his best, at home, he went everywhere carrying a small tank of oxygen. The surgery, a gastric bypass, went well, and he steadily improved. One day several months after the operation he came to see me without his usual oxygen tank. He explained that he no longer needed it, and that he was discharged from the care of the pulmonary doctors. At six months after surgery he had lost more than 100 pounds and he stopped seeing me at that time. I assume he feels so well that he doesn't think he needs me anymore. He's probably right.

Some of the other formerly Pickwickian patients have done so well that I completely forgot they ever had this condition. When I started to prepare this chapter, I surprisingly found their names on the list. I guess that's a measure of success, too.

I can sum up by emphasizing that the Pickwickian syndrome, or whatever you want to call it, is potentially a life-threatening and lethal condition. Aggressive treatment by dieting or antiobesity surgery is the answer and, when successful, results in a cure. From then on these individuals can lead normal lives.

The treatment of the Pickwickian syndrome was very successful. Patients were completely able to resume a normal life. This was very satisfying to the surgeon and all physicians managing these patients. The role of plastic surgery in the management of the very obese patient will be discussed in the next chapter.

23

The Role of Plastic Surgery

O, that this too too solid flesh would melt, thaw and resolve itself into a dew!

—Shakespeare, *Hamlet*

"Suppose I lose a lot of weight after the operation, what happens to all the extra skin?" This is one of the most common questions I am asked after I finish my one-hour discussion about gastric bypass with a new patient. I tell patients that, fortunately, as the weight is gradually lost, the skin shrinks down and nothing has to be done about it. But, there are some patients who do need some help, specifically the help of an experienced plastic surgeon. I have been fortunate in having colleagues who are superb plastic surgeons.*

INDICATIONS FOR PLASTIC SURGERY

About 20 percent of my patients have needed some form of plastic surgery. It's almost but not completely predictable which patients will need it. The heaviest patients are more likely to need plastic surgery, but this is not an absolute rule, and in some very big patients the skin retracts enough with the weight loss to be esthetically acceptable. Also, the older the patient is, the more likely the need will be for plastic surgery. Skin

---

*Dr. Jane Petro has helped me in the writing of this chapter.

elasticity decreases as we all get older. But again there have been exceptions. Finally, much does depend on where most of the fat deposits are located. Some had the so-called truncal obesity, where the abdomen is exceptionally large ("beer bellies"), and may already hang down toward the knees. Other patients have enormous thighs and buttocks without a huge abdomen. Still others are just very big all over.

As they lose weight, many patients ask if there is anything they could do to avoid the necessity for eventual plastic surgery. Specifically would exercise tighten this skin? Probably the real answer is that exercise cannot help the skin to retract and shrink. Although the muscles beneath the skin do contract during exercise, there are no muscles in the skin itself that can contract and tighten. Nevertheless, I never discourage patients from exercising. With exercise, the fat beneath the skin tends to decrease further, and also the fluid in the tissues beneath the skin decreases. This is important since an accumulation of fluid can be heavy enough to increase the pull of gravity downward, stretching the skin even further.

There are specific indications for plastic surgery after losing a lot of weight. First there is body image, the perception we have of what we look like. Many things influence this perception, including the appearance of one's friends and family, the current styles and fashions, one's expectations after weight loss, the age and sex of the patient, and so on. Some patients easily accept imperfections in their appearance. After all, with morbid obesity they have lived with worse imperfections for years. Others are more critical. They're looking for a new body without imperfections. Although this may be unrealistic, they still have their goals. They want sculpturing from plastic surgery, with "a little off here, a little off there, and a little off somewhere else." Their emotional well-being may be at stake, and this becomes a real challenge for the plastic surgeon.

PANNICULECTOMY

But there are some very legitimate physical health reasons that require plastic surgery. There are patients who have large amounts of excess skin, particularly in the abdominal area. It can actually hang down like a flap of extra skin. This is called a *panniculus*. There may be so much extra skin that it may hang all the way down to the knees, or even lower. I recently saw a picture of a patient who had a panniculus that nearly touched the floor. Serious problems can occur when the skin is folded on itself. It can be difficult to keep clean and dry, and the skin often rubs against itself continuously. This condition of irritation due to the rubbing of the skin against itself is called *intertrigo*. It can progress to a breakdown of the skin surface, or *ulceration*, bleeding, and serious infection. This certainly calls for surgical removal of the excess skin in an operation called a *panniculectomy* or *abdominoplasty*.

Another indication for this type of operation relates to the actual weight of the excess skin, which can be very heavy. I have had patients whose excess skin of the panniculus weighed 35 pounds when removed. The worst I have heard was a patient who had a panniculus that weighed 85 pounds. This weight concentrated in the abdomen can cause problems for the patient. The stretching and pulling can cause abdominal discomfort and pain. And there is a natural tendency for the back muscles to compensate for this extra weight in front by pulling back against the weight. This often causes considerable back pain in the upper and lower back areas. How would you feel if you had a 35-pound weight hanging down from your neck?

In addition, a large panniculus of the abdomen gets in the way of performing ordinary daily activities: walking, bending, turning, and stretching may be interfered with, and normal sexual function may be impossible.

A good case can be made for the use of plastic surgery of this type for these patients. The unfortunate thing is that many of the health-insurance companies refuse to cover it. When they hear "panniculectomy," they call it "cosmetic surgery," implying that it just is a frivolous desire of the patient to look more attractive. The plastic surgeons and I have spent much time trying to convince these companies that there are legitimate medical reasons for these operations, and we have offered to send photographs illustrating the problem. We are frequently turned down, and patients are told that they will have to assume all costs, including hospital bills, surgeons' fees, and so on.

This surgery must be planned carefully. It should be scheduled only when the weight loss has stopped and the new weight has stabilized. If the operation is done too early, and the patient continues to lose more weight, a second surgery might be necessary. Most surgeons feel that a panniculectomy should not be done at the time of the gastric bypass because the possibility of infection in the incision is too great. The incision for a panniculectomy is a very extensive one, and involves a lot of dissection. If the fat under the surface of this area were to become infected, it could be life threatening. The infection could be overwhelming involving such a vast area, and it would be difficult to treat.

There are no age limits for plastic surgery, and few medical reasons for limiting its use. Most of the patients needing this type of surgery have been women, but there have been some men as well.

There are several techniques for doing an abdominal panniculectomy, but the basic principle is the same. The excess skin and fat is cut out, and then the surgeon cuts underneath the skin (or "undermines" it) in order to make a flap of skin that can be pulled across or down to be stitched to the skin on the opposite side. This tightens up the remaining abdominal skin, relieves the symptoms, and results in a rather good appearance. The operation I've seen done most often by our plastic surgeons ends up with a long line of stitches across the very lowest part of the abdomen, the so-called bikini line. This generally heals very well, and sometimes the scar is not very apparent down in this area. It certainly gets well hidden under clothing or even swimwear.

I have made it sound very easy, but it really is a big operation since it involves considerable dissection of the abdominal wall tissue. Although the plastic surgeons use meticulous techniques, there sometimes can be a fair amount of blood loss. The skin, particularly when it hangs down, gets very swollen and heavy. Blood flow from the veins is fighting an uphill battle, literally, and the veins tend to enlarge and stretch. The first panniculectomy I watched on one of my patients, Lucy, was memorable. This was the patient who had a 35-pound panniculus. As the surgeons cut into the fat beneath the skin we saw a tubular structure wider than my thumb, and it had a dusky, dark reddish color. I couldn't figure out what it was. I suddenly had the horrible thought that the surgeons had gone deeper than expected, were now within the abdominal cavity, and the tubular structure was the intestine. With its color so dusky, I thought its blood supply was deficient and that it was becoming gangrenous. What a nightmare! But then I realized, it was just a hugely dilated vein in the fatty tissue beneath the skin, and that there were other veins nearby almost as large. By the way, not only did the specimen weigh 35 pounds, but it measured three square yards. This patient's panniculus hung down to her knees, and she complained that the sensation of the panniculus hitting against her knees was very unpleasant!

Another memorable panniculectomy involved one of my male patients who had lost almost 350 pounds as a result of his gastric bypass. He had a tremendous amount of excess skin also. When he was positioned on the operating table with the excess skin hanging down on both sides of him, it looked like he was melting away. Much excess skin was removed, which greatly improved his appearance.

Sometimes when the panniculus is exceptionally large, surgeons have pulled the panniculus up in the air, suspending it to overhead structures, such as pulleys attached to the ceiling, to make the removal a little easier. Pictures showing this look like some sort of medieval torture, but it is a good, effective technique (and, of course the anesthetized patient feels nothing).

There are complications that can occur with these operations, but fortunately they are very uncommon. Physicians are concerned that the edges of the skin stay healthy with a good blood supply. Sometimes part of the edges break down and slough off. This is not too serious and it still rapidly heals. Sometimes blood or clear serum can accumulate beneath the skin flaps, but gradually this drains to the outside or gets absorbed. The skin in this area may be numb for a while, with gradual return of feeling. But most patients do very well.

Patients often have more than one area of the body that needs corrective plastic surgery, and sometimes more than one area can be attended to in the same operation. The other areas most commonly needing plastic surgery are the upper arms, thighs, buttocks, and the breasts (for both men and women!).

UPPER ARMS

Flaps of skin hanging down from the upper arms are a particularly annoying problem. Some surgeons have called the excess skin "bat wings." Patients are very unhappy because they can't wear short-sleeved clothing and they may not be able to fit their arms comfortably into clothing with sleeves. At its worst, it is pretty unsightly. There are plastic surgery operations that can remove the excess skin. The only problem is that the long upper-arm scar remains visible even after complete healing. This is in contrast to the much more satisfactory scar seen after an abdominal panniculectomy. Patients are made aware of this before the surgeon does the procedure. In my opinion, the scar is far preferable to the unsightly bat-wing deformity.

THIGHS AND BUTTOCKS

After massive weight loss, some patients have problems resulting from excess skin folds in the thighs and buttocks. Again, you can almost always predict which patients may have this problem. In some, the predominance of weight seems to be in the thighs, way out of proportion to the rest of the body. If the weight loss results in sagging skin in the thigh area, patients may suffer from intertrigo and also have discomfort from clothing that fits well elsewhere in the body but tight around the thighs.

Plastic surgery can be helpful in treating the thigh and buttock areas, but, although improved, the results may not be everything the patient would hope. This can be a difficult part of the body to treat. An attempt is made to place the scars in the inner areas of the thighs where they will be less obvious. After the surgery, there may be some discomfort, even in sitting, but the result certainly does justify the discomfort.

BREASTS

The need for plastic surgery of the breasts after weight loss is much less common. For many women and men breast size decreases with the loss of body weight. But there are some who have large sagging breasts before surgery who don't experience the shrinkage and tightening up after weight loss. With some of these patients, intertrigo may develop, and if the breasts are heavy enough, neck and upper-back strain can occur. These patients are candidates for the plastic-surgery procedure called "reduction mammoplasty." Results are generally very satisfactory.

I've tried to point out that these plastic-surgery operations are necessary for the physical and medical health, as well as for the emotional health of the patients. The operations should be considered only for those who have a real need, and under these circumstances they should not be considered frivolous or merely cosmetic. Health-insurance carriers should understand this, and should provide adequate coverage.

LIPOSUCTION

Now let me say a few words about the relatively new procedure of liposuction. This has become the most commonly requested plastic-surgery procedure in America. But I have to emphasize that it is not, let me repeat, not an operation for relieving morbid obesity. The French surgeon who popularized liposuction, Dr. Gerard Illouz, emphasized that not more than

6 pounds of fat should be removed at a time. Now 6 pounds is not very much when you consider that morbidly obese individuals are at least 100 pounds over ideal weight. On the other hand, removal of the *bulk* that constitutes 6 pounds of fat can be very worthwhile. That is the value of liposuction. It can remove an area of fatty tissue that's causing localized bulging in an inappropriate part of the body.

In other words, liposuction is very useful for the person who has bulges on the outside of the upper thighs, sometimes called "saddlebags." In fact, this is probably the most common body site where liposuction is used. Other bulging deformities where this procedure is used include the sides of the lower abdomen ("love handles" or "hiprolls"), the inner thighs, the knees, the buttocks, and the "double-chin" area. It can be an effective operation on morbidly obese patients who have lost weight from gastric-stapling operations, but who have some localized areas, and the key word is *localized,* where inappropriate bulging is present. The operation is done for cosmetic purposes, and cannot be justified as being done for medical reasons.

The principle of the procedure is a simple one, namely the sucking out of fat in localized areas beneath the skin. It should only be done by trained, experienced surgeons. Success depends not only on the proper technique used, but also on the proper selection of patients. The patient's skin must be able to contract down after some of the underlying fat is removed so that the desired result can be attained. Ideally, younger patients, those under fifty, make the best candidates for this procedure, but older patients with good skin elasticity also may do well.

The operation is done under general anesthesia with the patient asleep. The area to be liposuctioned is first injected with saline, a salt solution. Some surgeons include a chemical called *hyaluronidase* which can help to spread the injected saline into the area. Others may add *epinephrine* (adrenaline) to the saline solution which tends to decrease the amount of bleeding under the skin. Then a very small incision, a quarter to half an inch long, is made, and the hollow metal suction rod is inserted into the fatty tissue under the skin. Before applying suction, a number of tunnels are made with the metal rod. Then the rod is attached by tubing to a suction machine, and the fat is sucked out as the rod is passed back and forth along the tunneled areas. Mostly fat is sucked out at first, but gradually some bleeding occurs, and the blood is also sucked out. The operations usually take less than one hour.

After the operation, patients may be instructed to wear a compressive binder or bandage to help in the healing. There may be some tenderness in the area of the liposuctioning, and sometimes some numbness for a while. Swelling and bruising of the skin is common, but it gradually disappears after several weeks. Patients are usually able to return to work after only a few days.

Complications from liposuction done by an experienced surgeon are uncommon, according to Mladick[1] and Gargan and Courtiss.[2] Occasionally some dimpling or waviness is seen after the procedure which may make the result less than ideal. Serious complications are rare. There have been a few deaths from infection, embolus to the lungs, and injuries to the abdominal organs, but these are fortunately very rare. But it is important to stress that this procedure must be performed by an experienced surgeon.

Reaccumulation of fat in the area that has undergone liposuction does not occur. But a small number of patients may need a second operation, as a sort of touchup, because of what appears to be insufficient removal of the fat at the first surgery.

Liposuction is a good cosmetic operation for the removal of localized areas of fat. It may be helpful to the former morbidly obese patient *after* weight loss, but is not a substitute for a weight-reducing gastric-bypass operation.

As you can see, there is a role for plastic surgeons in the management of the morbidly obese patient. Mostly, it involves the formerly obese person after he or she has lost considerable weight. With this chapter, the book is virtually complete, but the last two chapters are important since they deal with my comments about the surgery for the morbidly obese and comments from the patients themselves.

NOTES

1. R. Mladick, "Experience with the Illouz Technique of Lipoplasty in 1,000 Patients," *Contemporary Surgery* 34 (1989): 27–38.

2. T. J. Gargan and E. H. Courtiss, "The Risks of Suction Lipectomy," *Clinical Plastic Surgery* 11 (1984): 457–63.

24

Comments on the Surgery
for Morbid Obesity

All the fat shall be in the fire.
—Cervantes, *Don Quixote*

I have probably talked to more than a thousand people who fall in the category of morbid obesity, and have operated on about 750 of them. I think I have learned a great deal about them, and about their relationships with their families, friends, co-workers, and doctors. Many suffer from the frustrations of trying to lead a "normal" life in spite of their excessive obesity and their inability to lose weight by "ordinary" dietary means. They are often teased, ridiculed, criticized, and even attacked because of their dietary problems. They are discriminated against when choosing educational opportunities or seeking employment, and may be passed over for advancement in their workplace. They are less likely to be admitted to the better colleges, less likely to be hired for a job, and less likely to be promoted in their jobs.

As such, the significantly obese are probably the last group in America that is not adequately protected by law. They have no effective voice politically, although there apparently is a group called the National Association to Advance Fat Acceptance. There have been several recent court cases contesting alleged discrimination against very obese individuals. These cases included that of a young woman who was dismissed from a college's nursing program because of her "eating disorder" (she weighed more than 300 pounds) and an obese woman who was passed over for promotion at work. For many of the morbidly obese, their lives are not happy ones, and they see much of life passing by without their participation.

196

Gastric bypass is a good operation. Not perfect, but how many things are? Can it be further improved upon? I'm not sure. Could a better operation be developed? Sure, but at this point I don't see anything better. I have no doubt that someday there will be medication more effective than any operation for the treatment of morbid obesity. Appetite and satiation are complicated matters. When more is learned about the chemical reactions in the body that control appetite and satiation, a medical treatment of weight control should be feasible. I think it's inevitable, but the only question is when will we have this knowledge. It still could be a long way off.

Morbid obesity is a complicated matter, often controversial. There are some things related to it that make me very angry. Particularly, those people who say to me, "Why do you bother with these patients? They just refuse to use self-control to cut down on their eating. They're just not worth your efforts." Wouldn't it be ironic if scientists someday find definitively that the morbidly obese have some chemical imbalance, not necessarily hormonal, that prevents them from cutting down on their caloric intake? Or possibly that there is some genetic factor causing the whole thing, preventing them from dieting successfully? In the meantime, let's show some compassion for these unfortunate people who would like to be thin, in this thin world of ours.

Allow me some positive and negative comments about the world surrounding morbid obesity.

Families. The family members, husbands, wives, children, who are fully supportive, and who encourage the patient as the weight is being lost, are just wonderful. What a difference this makes to the patient! Then, on the other side, are the families who argue against having an operation even though they know nothing about it, and are unwilling to learn, even though the patient is crying out desperately for help. They're the ones who say "Just go home and diet," even though multitudes of diets already haven't worked. (And they're the ones who are ready to sue the hospital and doctors the moment there is any sort of a problem. All of a sudden they start to show great concern for the patient.)

Information Sources. The amount of misinformation about morbid obesity and the gastric bypass is incredible. Talk shows tend to sensationalize the whole thing, and continue to pass on incorrect information. The same goes for many of the magazine articles I've seen. There is no question about it, morbid obesity is a ripe subject for exploitation. But every so often it is refreshing to see a responsible, straightforward, accurate discussion of the subject in the printed media.

Physicians. I applaud the physicians who admit their frustrations in treating the very obese, and who are willing to learn about the newer surgical attempts to treat morbid obesity. I like it when a physician cares enough about his or her patient to have the patient seek appropriate surgical attention for the problem. I do not applaud the "just go home and diet" doctors, who show no understanding of the problem, or those who spread their own misinformation to the patient ("You will have terrible diarrhea" or "Don't you know how dangerous this is?"). I do not like the doctors who, when giving a "second opinion" requested by the insurance company, say "Yes, you need this operation, but I can do it better" or "I can send you to my friend who does it better." Very unethical and downright dishonest.

Nurses. I have seen hospital nurses who are just "against the whole thing" and don't want to understand why the patient needs an operation. I have seen anger and actual hostility against the patients. Happily, in time many of the nurses develop better relationships with the patients, particularly after they see some of the beneficial results of the weight loss. Most patients undergoing gastric bypass need good nursing care, emotional as well as physical support, and when there are nurses who give this kind of support, the treatment process goes much better.

Nutritionalists. The nutritionalists who are willing to learn about the surgery and the management of our patients are great. They can be very helpful and supportive both to doctors and to patients. But some of them don't want to understand or to work together, and may unintentionally give the patients wrong information. Some will say that what we are doing just can't work, in spite of our experience with hundreds and thousands of patients. Education helps, and as they see the patients before and after the surgery, an understanding does develop.

Health-Insurance Providers. I applaud the companies that have learned that surgical treatment of obesity is effective in terms of improving the health of the patients, and is also cost effective in terms of actually saving money for their companies. There are other companies that continually put roadblocks in our way before they are willing to approve the surgery for the patients. How many times have I had to write letters explaining that this is not cosmetic surgery, and then had to send the letters again months later because the companies have misplaced the originals? Or they misplace operative reports, pathology reports, etc., that have been sent to them. Then there are the companies that agree that the patient must be hospitalized for the surgery, but cannot guarantee payment until they reevaluate it *after* the surgery is done. And there are still companies that refuse to approve these operations in spite of universal agreement that they have become the treatment of choice for morbidly obese people who have failed attempts to diet. I am optimistic that this situation will improve.

Patients. Most of them are excited with the prospects of being operated on, and losing weight. Many are nervous about it, and that's understandable. Most are very cooperative and comply with our instructions. Some patients are difficult, uncooperative, and make everything needlessly complicated. In time most concerns are resolved. Most patients are very pleased with the results. A very high percent of my new patients have been referred to me by others who have already had the surgery and are happy with their new life.

25

In the Patients' Own Words

I have read your glorious letters,
Where you threw aside all fetters,
Spoke your thoughts and mind out freely
In your own delightful style.
—Bessie Chandler, *Letter to Mrs. Thomas Carlyle*

Throughout the years I have been doing this type of surgery I have received many letters and cards from patients. Some have been complaints about one thing or another, but more often the letters have reflected the pleasure and delight in what has occurred since their operations. The letters have varied from those that are well written and articulate to others hurriedly scribbled on a scrap piece of paper. But in most letters, the message is clear. Life is better!

I thought the most appropriate way of ending this book is to let the patients have the last word. I have picked some excerpts from recent letters that I thought were especially interesting.

One of the most interesting letters was sent to me from a patient who originally had a jejunoileal bypass many years ago in Syracuse. His single-spaced letter went on for five pages. (He wrote that his wife would not type any more than this.) Let me quote a few parts.

"My life was affected greatly! I went from a preoperative weight of 444 pounds to a relatively stable 220 pounds for most of the postoperative years. . . . My self-image greatly improved. I could buy clothes in my new size almost anywhere, in a great variety of styles and colors. I could wear blue jeans and find them to fit. I went from a size 22-23 shirt, 66-inch waist pants to a man's 16-16½ shirt and 40-42 pants. I could fit comfortably in even small-size cars. I purchased a Toyota Celica, which would not have been possible earlier.

"I had always been obese, weighing over 200 pounds in sixth grade, 330 pounds at high school graduation, and I can never remember a time when my weight wasn't increasing. . . . Although I was always obese, I was active in sports, swimming, dating, and most juvenile activities throughout my high school and college years. Dating was not a problem, except for finding a long-term relationship that might lead to marriage. It obviously would take a special person to overlook my weight problem.

"Eventually with my new self (physical) I met my future wife, while on a trip to France in the summer of 1979. Although we only had a casual friendship at that time, one year later, I saw her again and love struck eventually leading to marriage. She knew about my bypass operation, and of course never knew me during my morbid-obese years. She has seen pictures of me from this time and I believe this would have made a difference in her accepting my proposal.

"Sometime in the spring or early summer of 1975, I saw a television program which treated the subject of obesity and focused on a man who had undergone the J-I intestinal-bypass surgery. After a consultation with my family doctor, he advised me to contact your office in Syracuse, which as you know led to my eventual surgery in 1975.

"During the fifteen or so months after surgery, the amazing success and positive reinforcement that I received really built up my confidence and ego. A lot was happening, a new image, new expectations, but still a lot of loneliness beneath it all. I had dated several people during this time but nothing lasting really occurred. I was looking but not finding. I probably could have taken advantage of my new circumstances and bar-hopped looking for one-night stands, or short-term relationships for temporary physical satisfaction, but not only would that not have satisfied my needs and desires, it would have betrayed a trust and prayer, and indeed a conviction that I had made to God weeks before my surgery. And that was that if the surgery weight loss were successful, I did not want it to lead towards a life that took advantage of others for my own personal pleasure, but rather towards positive worthwhile commitments that would be hopefully forever. God has never let me down! He has always been with me and led me towards the right choices, whenever and wherever they have shown up. Most of all when I was on the trip to France. It was on this trip that I eventually met my wife. . . .

"Our first child was born January 25, 1983, and our son was born December 3, 1987, and my million-dollar family became a reality.

"From 1975 until June of 1992, I have had almost all positive results from the bypass operation. Very few foods had given me any problems. I had enjoyed many health benefits—very low cholesterol, triglycerides, blood sugar, etc. . . . I usually took vitamins and, except for the constant diarrhea 4 or 5 times a day, I had no major complaints. Many times I have been asked if I had to do it over again would I . . . ? My answer has always been yes, with some qualifications. If I had been as some of your early patients were and only lost fifty pounds or so, I probably would not have gone through everything that I did a second or third time. But I never had to cross that bridge. Until June of 1992, which brings us to the reattachment of the intestine and the stomach bypass. Once again, I found myself both in God's care and your hands, Dr. Ackerman. Once again, I have not been disappointed. The first month was hard. But the ongoing adjustments are both tolerable and rewarding. My weight is presently 215-220, although my home scales show 210."

The patient concludes his letter with an anecdote that is typical of many reported to me by my patients. I quote again.

"During my senior year at Penn State I had a roommate in an off-campus apartment, named Mike. . . . I eventually became the best man at his wedding in the early 70s. As frequently happens, we got out of touch over the years and he hadn't seen me from about 1971 or 1972 until about 1978 or 1979. Only infrequent cards (birth of their child, Christmas, etc.) took place until one summer when I found myself in his hometown and wanted to look him up and surprise him, as I had done to many others, most of whom were taken aback and astonished, but soon recognized me. Not so with Mike.

"I went to his parents' home and asked if Mike was around and his dad gave me directions to a picnic where he was. So I made my way to this picnic, found Mike working over a barbecue grill, and tapped him on the shoulder. I asked him if he could direct me to a local address which was in the area but I couldn't find. I played this routine with him, playing ignorance of his directions, and he even asked some friends for some help to count red lights and prospective turns, etc. Finally, I offered him my hand to thank him for taking so much time for a stranger, a passerby who was not familiar with the area and who needed help. But I kept his hand a little longer than usual and would not let it go, even when time became a little uncomfortable for both of us, and I squeezed it a little harder, continuing to thank him for his kindness and refusing to let him withdraw his hand from mine. I could tell that he was very uncomfortable with this. And I was enjoying every second. After about one and a half minutes, I said I can't believe how ignorant you really are—that you could talk to me for the better part of 12-15 minutes, have a prolonged handshake to the point of wondering who this strange guy was, and not recognize the guy who was the best man at his own wedding! Needless to say, he looked about as astonished as anything and couldn't believe his own eyes!! I had played this game with others at high school reunions and such, but never with the success that I did with Mike.

"I am again in hurried circumstances as my family and I are leaving for eleven days at Disney World. . . . I expect to do most things at Disney World, with the exception of bungee jumping, which I would not do for love or money!"

With his letter he enclosed some incredible before and after pictures. By the way, he is in error. My first patients did *not* only lose fifty pounds or so.

Let me move on to excerpts from another letter, this time from a young woman who underwent a gastric bypass. She writes:

"My weight has changed my life in so many ways. Prior to my weight loss I was very self-conscious and insecure about myself. I had a three-year-old at the time and my weight prevented me from being comfortable enough with myself to be seen outside playing with my son. I knew that if my son was going to grow up being extroverted and enjoying himself then I would need to change. Losing weight was just the change I needed.

"Since the weight loss a lot of things have happened. . . . I knew that if things didn't change, my son would grow up sheltered because of *my* insecurities. And that's no way to raise a child. He is now six years old and a very happy extroverted child.

"My weight loss has changed my life in almost a domino-like effect. I'm so secure and happy with myself. It's such a good feeling to be one of the 'normal,' and not an outsider. Of course having a choice of clothing styles to wear is a plus.

"We recently sold our house and moved up north. I would never have even thought about this change if I had still been fat. We moved from a place where everyone knew me the way I was, to a place where we didn't know a soul. First impressions are very important and hard to cope with when you're fat. Your size is just the first thing that people notice, or so you think.

"After the move, I started a new job. Every day on a new job you meet so many new people who now take you for what you do and how you do it, instead of what you look like.

"And I'm very happy to say that between the changes above, came my greatest joy. I had a baby five months ago. I have a history of infertility. My son, now six, was conceived when I was fat. At that time I needed to be treated with Clonid in order to conceive. I tried again to conceive on Clonid therapy without luck, while I was still fat.

"What a surprise for us to find out last summer that I was pregnant. It happened just naturally, like most other couples in the world. No test tubes, blood tests, temperature taking, etc. I have no doubt in my mind that if I was still fat, my son would not be here now.

"I almost neglected to tell you that we went on vacation after selling the house. We went to Cancun, Mexico. I wasn't embarrassed at all to be seen in a bathing suit. We went on catamaran rides, went snorkeling, and I learned to scuba dive. It was *fantastic!* I certainly would not have gone to Cancun and would have missed the experience of a lifetime going scuba diving if I was still fat."

She also enclosed photos of herself, although she said it was hard to find "before" pictures. She never wanted to have her picture taken. Now, she said, in the pictures other people hide behind her, instead of the other way around.

In other letters I have received, even more anger is expressed about how the world treats people who have major weight problems. Let me quote from a letter written by another woman who had a gastric bypass:

"Before my operation I was a FAT person with very little self-esteem and confidence. I was a thin person in my heart and soul who could not find the way out.

"People are extremely prejudiced towards fat people. I was passed over for employment positions because of my size. For example, I was eighteen years old and weighed in at 211 pounds. I had an interview with a large corporation in Manhattan. The personnel agent told me I was not suited for the position and that before I interview again in the city that I should lose some serious weight. She told me appearances are everything, if you look sloppy they base your working habits on your appearance. Being overweight is not businesslike. Over the years I blossomed to over 300 pounds. People tend to ignore you when you are overweight and those that do not ignore you usually are making a nasty or 'helpful' comment like why don't you lose some weight, you'll feel so much better.

Like any fat person chooses to be 300 pounds, like it was a goal we strive to reach.

"I work with people in the same office for seven years now and there are some of these people who never acknowledged my existence until I lost my weight. Now these same people invite me to social functions with them. I have told them that I am the same person I was before, just less of me, but they say that I was a very intimidating person, they said I was not as friendly as now. I would say I have to agree because I now have the confidence and self-esteem I never had before.

"I now have so much more energy, I take nice long walks, work out at the gym and at home, play on a softball team, etc.!!! When I go shopping I don't have to drive around and around waiting for a space to open up to be able to park close to the door, and when I go inside to shop I don't have to buy all the junk food the place has to offer. I can now walk into the ice cream shoppe in my town without people staring at me and wondering why is this fat person eating this, go home and eat carrot sticks. We all know these people do think these things and some of them even have the ———— to say it to your face.

"When I decided to have this surgery I went on a quest for information, speaking to surgeons, reading information pamphlets, and speaking to persons who already had the surgery . . . . My husband was very supportive of my decision and we finally set the date. It is all over now and I have lost more weight than I weigh right now. I would never have been able to do this without this surgery. I began diets practically at birth, I can remember being on diet pills starting when I was in the third grade and as the years went on every diet out there was shoved in my face. The more I was forced to diet the more weight I gained. What an emotional roller coaster we are forced to live when overweight."

She concludes with a handwritten postscript saying, "We all should go on Oprah or Phil Donahue and let others out there know that this is available and that it *does* work."

The last letter I'll quote from was written by one of my older female patients who recently had a gastric bypass and then plastic surgery for her excessive abdominal-wall skin. She expresses lucidly what the weight loss has meant to her.

"I truly believed that I harbored a great anger at the knowledge that I should deny myself food. This just caused me to eat all the more. The surgery took that decision out of my hands! It just isn't possible for me to eat as I used to, but, and this is important, I can eat almost anything I feel like trying, instead of denying myself or feeling guilty if I do try something. The anger is gone. Remember, I was so depressed and suicidal that it was suggested that I attend HIP Mental Health Program. Although I still attend the group sessions, it is with a different attitude—happier and relaxed. Everyone commented re my improved appearance.

"My walk is better, I can bend and pick up dropped articles, instead of having to bring a chair over, sit down, and lean over to pick up. I have just returned from a visit to Windham, New York, to visit my granddaughter—I took AMTRAK! Since I've been practically a shut-in for a few years this trip was just like a trip to Europe for me. As you probably have guessed I am still overweight but I am losing a few pounds slowly and I rarely weigh in because it is not on my mind. I must state that the 'tummy tuck surgery' has also worked wonders. I am wearing dresses that I bought in San Diego ten years ago. I have a lap—I can put a dinner napkin on my lap! It stays and doesn't fall off. You just can't understand how I *hated* that ugly dropped abdomen flap hanging. Now it's gone. My skirts or dresses hang loose. I do not need a jacket or sweater to try and cover the flab.

"I am truly a happier person. I was realistic from the start. I wanted to be mentally and physically healthier. I think that has happened."

There are lots of other letters. One man reported that people can't tell him from his son, and that they both wear the same size clothes. Another said that he thinks he looks like a movie star, and that customers in the cafe where he works keep asking for the big guy who used to work there. Many report feeling twenty years younger, running up and down stairs, with unbelievable energy. Some have mentioned improvements in their employment status, back to work and no longer on disability and welfare. The majority of patients appear pleased with their "new" selves, and this is clearly reflected in the letters I have received.

Appendix

My Criteria for Operations
for Morbid Obesity

1. Patients must be morbidly obese. They should be one hundred pounds over ideal weight, or two times ideal weight. This obesity should have been present for at least five years.

2. A reasonable attempt to diet should have been made. The exact type of diet is less important.

3. Corrective endocrine problems causing the obesity should be ruled out by appropriate testing. Hypothyroidism and overactivity of the adrenal are most common. Hypothalamic injury can cause obesity, but it is not correctable.

4. Patients should represent a reasonable operative risk. Recent myocardial infarcts and severe pulmonary disease are serious problems affecting operative risk. Patients with Pickwickian syndrome (obese hypoventilation syndrome) pose serious risks, but the possible beneficial effects from surgery make the risk worthwhile.

5. The presence of obesity-related medical problems are not contraindications since they may improve or resolve with obesity surgery. These problems include diabetes, hypertension, Pickwickian syndrome, degenerative arthritis, and obesity-related emotional problems. However, these are not considered a requirement for surgery.

6. Patients must be able to understand the operation, to follow directions, to take medications when ordered, and to keep postoperative appointments.

7. Patients must be in the age range from the teens to sixty-five years.

Glossary

Anthropometry. The study and technique of human body measurement.

Bile. A bitter, alkaline greenish or brownish-yellow liquid that is secreted by the liver, stored in the gallbladder, and discharged into the **duodenum**, and that aids in digestion by saponification of fats.

Duodenum. The first part of the small intestine, 8 to 10 inches long. It contains the openings through which the pancreas and the bile drain.

Endoscopy. Examination of the interior of a hollow organ, such as the stomach, using a special tube fitted with a lens and a light source.

Endotracheal tube. A tube passed through the mouth into the trachea, used for assisting breathing.

Gastric bypass. Weight-reduction operation, with small stomach pouch and a narrow emptying outlet made to the intestine. Most of the stomach and **duodenum** are bypassed.

Gastrojejunostomy. Surgical creation of a connection between the stomach and **jejunum**.

Gastroplasty. Weight-reduction operation, with small stomach pouch emptying through a narrow outlet directly to the lower part of the stomach.

Hernia. The protrusion of a body structure through the wall that normally contains it. Frequently involving the abdominal wall.

Ileum. The lower portion of the small intestine, extending from the **jejunum** to the large intestine.

Intestinal bypass. Same as the **jejunoileal bypass**.

Jejunum. The midportion of the small intestine, extending from the **duodenum** to the **ileum**.

Jejunocolic bypass. Obsolete weight-reduction operation, connecting the upper part of the small intestine to the large intestine, bypassing most of the small intestine and part of the large intestine.

Jejunoileal bypass. Weight-reduction operation, connecting the upper part of the small intestine to the lower part, bypassing about 90 percent of the midpart of the small intestine.

Leptin. A hormone that causes the body to eat less and to shed weight. (Most of the studies have been on obese mice).

Liposuction. Plastic-surgery procedure, consisting of the sucking out of fat in localized areas beneath the skin.

Morbid obesity. People who are at least 100 pounds over their ideal weight, who already have, or are likely to develop, major medical or physical problems relating to their weight.

Nasogastric tube. A tube, inserted through the nose, down the esophagus, into the stomach. Put on suction, it is used for emptying the contents of the stomach.

Panniculectomy. Plastic-surgery operation, with surgical removal of excess skin and fat hanging down from the abdominal wall. Also called *abdominoplasty*.

Peritonitis. Inflammation of the peritoneum (the lining of the walls of the abdominal cavity), usually severe.

Pickwickian syndrome. Condition including **morbid obesity**, respiratory difficulties, disturbance of normal sleeping patterns, retained carbon dioxide, and decreased oxygen in the blood. Also called *obese hypoventilation syndrome*.

Prader-Willi syndrome. Condition including uncontrolled overeating with massive weight gain, short stature, some mental retardation, retarded sexual development, and temper tantrums.

Stoma. An opening. A term, used by surgeons, to denote the opening made surgically between two parts of the gastrointestinal tract.

Syndrome. A group of symptoms and signs, which, when considered together, characterize a disease.

Trachea. Windpipe; connection from throat to lungs.

Tracheotomy. The procedure of cutting into the **trachea** through the neck, usually to make breathing easier.

Triglycerides. Fatty substances found in the bloodstream. Along with cholesterol constitutes serum lipids.

Index

213